Anesthesiologists in Times of Disaster

Editors

JESSE RAITEN
LEE A. FLEISHER

ANESTHESIOLOGY CLINICS

www.anesthesiology.theclinics.com

Consulting Editor
LEE A. FLEISHER

June 2021 • Volume 39 • Number 2

ELSEVIER

1600 John F. Kennedy Boulevard • Suite 1800 • Philadelphia, Pennsylvania, 19103-2899

http://www.theclinics.com

ANESTHESIOLOGY CLINICS Volume 39, Number 2
June 2021 ISSN 1932-2275, ISBN-13: 978-0-323-81347-1

Editor: Joanna Collett
Developmental Editor: Arlene Campos

Anesthesiology Clinics (ISSN 1932-2275) is published quarterly by Elsevier Inc., 360 Park Avenue South, New York, NY 10010-1710. Months of issue are March, June, September, and December. Periodicals postage paid at New York, NY and at additional mailing offices. Subscription prices are $100.00 per year (US student/resident), $368.00 per year (US individuals), $455.00 per year (Canadian individuals), $957.00 per year (US institutions), $1000.00 per year (Canadian institutions), $100.00 per year (Canadian student/resident), $225.00 per year (foreign student/resident), $488.00 per year (foreign individuals), and $1000.00 per year (foreign institutions). To receive student and resident rate, orders must be accompanied by name of affiliated institution, date of term, and the *signature* of program/residency coordinator on institutions letterhead. Orders will be billed at individual rate until proof of status is received. Foreign air speed delivery is included in all *Clinics'* subscription prices. All prices are subject to change without notice. POSTMASTER: Send address changes to *Anesthesiology Clinics,* Elsevier Health Sciences Division, Subscription Customer Service, 3251 Riverport Lane, Maryland Heights, MO 63043. Customer Service (orders, claims, online, change of address): Elsevier Health Sciences Division, Subscription Customer Service, 3251 Riverport Lane, Maryland Heights, MO 63043. **Tel:1-800-654-2452 (U.S. and Canada); 314-447-8871 (outside U.S. and Canada). Fax: 314-447-8029. E-mail: journalscustomerservice-usa@elsevier.com (for print support); journalsonlinesupport-usa@elsevier.com (for online support)**.

Reprints. For copies of 100 or more of articles in this publication, please contact the Commercial Reprints Department, Elsevier Inc., 360 Park Avenue South, New York, NY 10010-1710. Tel.: 212-633-3874; Fax: 212-633-3820; E-mail: reprints@elsevier.com.

Anesthesiology Clinics, is also published in Spanish by McGraw-Hill Inter-americana Editores S. A., P.O. Box 5-237, 06500 Mexico D. F., Mexico.

Anesthesiology Clinics, is covered in *MEDLINE/PubMed (Index Medicus), Current Contents/Clinical Medicine, Excerpta Medica, ISI/BIOMED*, and *Chemical Abstracts.*

Contributors

CONSULTING EDITOR

LEE A. FLEISHER, MD, FACC, FAHA
Robert D. Dripps Professor and Chair of Anesthesiology and Critical Care, Professor of Medicine, Perelman School of Medicine, University of Pennsylvania, Philadelphia, Pennsylvania, USA

EDITORS

JESSE RAITEN, MD
Department of Anesthesiology and Critical Care, Perelman School of Medicine, University of Pennsylvania, Philadelphia, Pennsylvania, USA

LEE A. FLEISHER, MD, FACC, FAHA
Robert D. Dripps Professor and Chair of Anesthesiology and Critical Care, Professor of Medicine, Perelman School of Medicine, University of Pennsylvania, Philadelphia, Pennsylvania, USA

AUTHORS

SUBHASH P. ACHARYA, MD, FACC, FCCP
Professor, Department of Anaesthesiology, Tribhuvan University Teaching Hospital, Maharajgunj, Kathmandu, Nepal

BROOKE ALBRIGHT-TRAINER, MD, FASA
Assistant Professor, Former Major, MC, USAF and CCAT Director for 10th EAEF, Department of Anesthesiology, Division of Critical Care Medicine, University of Virginia Health System, Charlottesville, Virginia, USA; Department of Anesthesiology, Central Virginia VA Health Care System, Richmond, Virginia, USA

ASHISH AMATYA, MD
Anesthesiologist and Head, Department of Cardiac Anaesthesiology and Critical Care, Shahid Gangalal National Heart Center, Kathmandu, Nepal

GIACOMO BELLANI, MD, PhD
Department of Medicine and Surgery, University of Milano-Bicocca, Department of Emergency and Intensive Care, San Gerardo Hospital, Monza, Italy

CHESTER BUCKENMAIER III, MS, MD
Professor, Anesthesiology, Uniformed Services University, Bethesda, Maryland, USA

XIANGDONG CHEN, MD, PhD
Department of Anesthesiology, Institute of Anesthesia and Critical Care Medicine, Union Hospital, Tongji Medical College, Huazhong University of Science and Technology, Wuhan, Hubei, China

XUEYIN CHEN, MD
Department of Anesthesiology, Institute of Anesthesia and Critical Care Medicine, Union Hospital, Tongji Medical College, Huazhong University of Science and Technology, Wuhan, Hubei, China

TSUI SIN YUI CINDY, MBBS
Clinical Assistant Professor (Honorary), Department of Anaesthesia and Intensive Care, The Chinese University of Hong Kong, Prince of Wales Hospital, Shatin New Territories, Hong Kong

REAR ADMIRAL DARIN VIA, MD
Trauma Anesthesiologist, Commander, Naval Medical Forces Atlantic, Portsmouth, Virginia, USA; Clinical Professor, Uniformed Services University of Health Sciences, Bethesda, Maryland, USA

EMILY GORDON, MD, MSEd
Vice Chair of Education and Program Director, Department of Anesthesiology and Critical Care, Hospital of the University of Pennsylvania, Philadelphia, Pennsylvania, USA

GIACOMO GRASSELLI, MD
Department of Pathophysiology and Transplantation, University of Milan, Department of Anesthesia, Intensive Care and Emergency, Fondazione IRCCS Ca' Granda Ospedale Maggiore Policlinico, Milan, Italy

JONATHAN HASTIE, MD
Department of Anesthesiology, Columbia University Irving Medical Center, New York, New York, USA

KONSTANTIN INOZEMTSEV, MD
Department of Anesthesiology, Dartmouth-Hitchcock Medical Center, Lebanon, New Hampshire, USA

J. MICHAEL JAEGER, PhD, MD
Emeritus Associate Professor, Former Surgeon General, Joint Special Operations Air Detachment-Arabian Peninsula, Departments of Anesthesiology and Surgery, Division of Critical Care Medicine, University of Virginia Health System, Charlottesville, Virginia, USA

RITESH LAMSAL, MD, DM
Assistant Professor, Department of Anaesthesiology, Tribhuvan University Teaching Hospital, Maharajgunj, Kathmandu, Nepal

MEGHAN LANE-FALL, MD, MSHP
Department of Anesthesiology and Critical Care, Perelman School of Medicine, University of Pennsylvania, Philadelphia, Pennsylvania, USA

RENYU LIU, MD, PhD
Department of Anesthesiology and Critical Care, Perelman School of Medicine, University of Pennsylvania, Center of Penn Global Health Scholar, Professor, Philadelphia, Pennsylvania, USA

DEREK NICHOLAS LODICO, DO
Cardiothoracic and Trauma Anesthesiologist, Commander, Naval Trauma Training Command, Los Angeles County + University of Southern California Medical Center, Keck School of Medicine of USC, Los Angeles, California, USA; Assistant Professor, Uniformed Services University of Health Sciences, Bethesda, Maryland, USA

YING HUI LOW, MD
Department of Anesthesia, Critical Care and Pain Medicine, Massachusetts General Hospital, Harvard Medical School, Boston, Massachusetts, USA

BAJRACHARYA SMRITI MAHAJU, MD
Registrar Anesthesiologist, Department of Cardiac Anaesthesiology and Critical Care, Shahid Gangalal National Heart Center, Kathmandu, Nepal

AURORA MAGLIOCCA, MD, PhD
Department of Medicine and Surgery, University of Milano-Bicocca, Monza, Italy

VANESSA MAZANDI, MD
Pediatric Critical Care Medicine Fellow, Department of Anesthesiology and Critical Care, Children's Hospital of Philadelphia, Philadelphia, Pennsylvania, USA

ALEXANDER NAGREBETSKY, MD, MSc
Department of Anesthesia, Critical Care and Pain Medicine, Massachusetts General Hospital, Harvard Medical School, Boston, Massachusetts, USA

OLIVER PANZER, MD
Department of Anesthesiology, Columbia University Irving Medical Center, New York, New York, USA

ANTONIO PESENTI, MD
Department of Pathophysiology and Transplantation, University of Milan, Department of Anesthesia, Intensive Care and Emergency, Fondazione IRCCS Ca' Granda Ospedale Maggiore Policlinico, Milan, Italy

JESSE RAITEN, MD
Department of Anesthesiology and Critical Care, Perelman School of Medicine, University of Pennsylvania, Philadelphia, Pennsylvania, USA

EMANUELE REZOAGLI, MD, PhD
Department of Medicine and Surgery, University of Milano-Bicocca, Department of Emergency and Intensive Care, San Gerardo Hospital, Monza, Italy

DARIAN C. RICE, MD, PhD
Associate Professor, Department of Anesthesiology, Division of Critical Care Medicine, University of Virginia Health System, Charlottesville, Virginia, USA; Former Head of Anesthesiology and Critical Care, Kandahar Air Field Role 3 Multinational Medical Unit, Afghanistan

LUDMILLA CANDIDO SANTOS, MD
Emergency Medicine Network, Massachusetts General Hospital, Harvard Medical School, Boston, Massachusetts, USA

MICHAEL SCOTT, MB ChB
Department of Anesthesiology and Critical Care, Perelman School of Medicine, University of Pennsylvania, Philadelphia, Pennsylvania, USA

GENTLE S. SHRESTHA, MD, FACC, EDIC, FCCP, FNCS
Associate Professor, Department of Anaesthesiology, Tribhuvan University Teaching Hospital, Maharajgunj, Kathmandu, Nepal

RANISH SHRESTHA, BS
Microbiologist, Infection Control Unit, Nepal Cancer Hospital and Research Center, Lalitpur, Nepal

MAC STABEN, MD, MA
Department of Anesthesiology and Critical Care, Perelman School of Medicine, University of Pennsylvania, Philadelphia, Pennsylvania, USA

PRADIP TIWARI, MD, FACC
Consultant Intensivist, Department of Critical Care, Norvic International Hospital, Thapathali, Kathmandu, Nepal

ROBERT VIETOR III, MD
Assistant Professor, Anesthesiology, Uniformed Services University, Bethesda, Maryland, USA

GEBHARD WAGENER, MD
Department of Anesthesiology, Columbia University Irving Medical Center, New York, New York, USA

DAVID S. WANG, MD
Department of Anesthesiology, Columbia University Irving Medical Center, New York, New York, USA

JING WU, MD, PhD
Department of Anesthesiology, Institute of Anesthesia and Critical Care Medicine, Union Hospital, Tongji Medical College, Huazhong University of Science and Technology, Wuhan, Hubei, China

SHANGLONG YAO, MD, PhD
Department of Anesthesiology, Institute of Anesthesia and Critical Care Medicine, Union Hospital, Tongji Medical College, Huazhong University of Science and Technology, Wuhan, Hubei, China

Contents

Events during the 2020 COVID-19 pandemic have demonstrated how disasters can disrupt the flow of health care delivery. Disaster events may become more common, and health care providers need proper training in how to manage patients affected by these events. Literature from anesthetic management from prior disasters, other specialties, and low-income and middle-income countries, offers guidance for how to respond to disasters. An effective disaster response requires a comprehensive plan that is rehearsed and well executed. Health care workers responding to a disaster may suffer physical and psychological consequences.

This article documents experiences from frontline anesthesia providers in Wuhan, China, mainly from the anesthesiologists in Union Hospital, Tongji Medical College, Huazhong University of Science and Technology, Wuhan, Hubei, China. Those experiences offer valuable insight into the processes used to optimize the emergency response system, and the medical resources and emergency allocation, as well as providing information on the role anesthesiologists played in managing the pandemic.

Italy was the first western country facing an outbreak of coronavirus disease 2019 (COVID-19). The first Italian patient diagnosed with COVID-19 was admitted, on Feb. 20, 2020, to the intensive care unit (ICU) in Codogno (Lodi, Lombardy, Italy), and the number of reported positive cases increased to 36 in the next 24 hours, and then exponentially for 18 days. This triggered a response that resulted in a massive surge in ICU bed capacity. The COVID19 Lombardy Network organized a structured logistic response and provided scientific evidence to highlight information on COVID-19 associated respiratory failure.

This article addresses the importance of anesthesiologists providing regional anesthesia techniques that are beneficial to the care of trauma patients in the field. It also discusses the advantages and risks associated with regional anesthesia in the field along with how to avoid those risks. In addition, it describes some of the benefits of modern ultrasound techniques compared with landmark techniques with stimulation and other important considerations when performing regional anesthesia in the field. The article gives the unique indications, risks, and key points of the most useful regional techniques for anesthesiologists operating in field environments.

COVID-19 challenged many facets of medicine. At the frontlines of managing the health care of the infected were anesthesiologists and critical care physicians, especially those in large cities. The Hospital of the University of Pennsylvania [HUP] was no exception. Through simulations, online education platforms, and most importantly creative scheduling that allows acquisition of skills and ACGME milestones to be met, COVID-19 allowed the Department of Anesthesiology and Critical Care at HUP to meet the challenges presented during the surge and create a template for future challenges to the US health care system.

In March 2020, the COVID-19 pandemic reached New York City, resulting in thousands of deaths over the following months. Because of the exponential spread of disease, the New York City hospital systems became rapidly overwhelmed. The Department of Anesthesiology at New York Presbyterian (NYP)-Columbia continued to offer anesthesia services for obstetrics and emergency surgery, while redirecting the rest of its staff to the expanded airway management role and the creation of the largest novel intensive care unit in the NYP system. Tremendous innovation and optimization were necessary in the face of material, physical, and staffing constraints.

The COVID-19 pandemic has seen many hurdles to crucial research processes, in particular those that depend on personnel interactions, in providing safeguards against the incipient infectious disease. At the same time, there was a rapid redirection of research, driven by popular and social media and demand for pandemic-related content, to the detriment of non–COVID-19 research and perhaps to COVID-19 research itself. This article provides historical context to research redirection and discusses approaches to optimizing research methodology in the setting of COVID-19 pandemic.

ANESTHESIOLOGY CLINICS

SERIES OF RELATED INTEREST

Critical Care Clinics

THE CLINICS ARE AVAILABLE ONLINE!
Access your subscription at:
www.theclinics.com

Preface

Anesthesiologists in Times of Disaster: A Rich History, a Busy Future

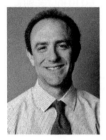
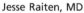
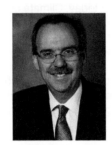

Jesse Raiten, MD Lee A. Fleisher, MD, FACC, FAHA
Editors

When the COVID-19 pandemic struck the United States in the early months of 2020, our national health care system was thrust into one of the most challenging periods it has faced in recent history. Over the ensuing months, millions of people fell ill, and hundreds of thousands died. Hospital facilities, particularly critical care resources, were stretched to capacity and beyond. It has been said that necessity is the mother of invention, and novel strategies and staffing paradigms were developed to not only provide medical care to patients but also maximize staff utilization and provide additional support where needed.

The health care community's response to COVID-19 was a tremendous team effort, bringing together professionals from every specialty and service. It comes as no surprise that anesthesiologists and anesthesia providers assumed central roles in the response, not only in the United States but also on a global scale. Anesthesiologists assumed care for critically ill patients on ventilators, developed novel strategies to safely intubate patients, led procedure teams, assisted overworked respiratory therapists, and provided critical council to hospital administrators as clinical landscapes radically shifted to accommodate a new patient population.

The role of anesthesiologists in times of disaster has a rich history, from the battlefields of World War II to the field hospitals and make-shift operating rooms that have accompanied virtually every natural disaster in recent times. Anesthesiologists, by virtue of their broad training in the care of critically ill patients, wide range of procedural skills, and proficiency with patient triage and risk assessment, are well suited to lead institutional and regional medical efforts in times of crisis.

In this issue of *Anesthesiology Clinics*, authors explore the vast roles that anesthesiologists play in times of disaster. We consider the fundamental requirements for a

Anesthesiology Clin 39 (2021) xi–xii
https://doi.org/10.1016/j.anclin.2021.03.005
1932-2275/21/© 2021 Published by Elsevier Inc.

anesthesiology.theclinics.com

successful disaster response plan, be it to respond to a natural or manmade disaster. A diverse group of authors from across the globe, including both developed and resource-limited countries, describes how they handled the COVID-19 pandemic, from China to Italy to Nepal. We then take an in-depth look at how anesthesiologists can lead in times of physical disasters, as well as in the unique environments of mass casualty events, war zones, and military special operations. Recognizing that health care systems have many mandates apart from direct patient care, we explore how resident education, as well as research activities, may be influenced and modified in times of calamity.

There are many threats facing the world today. Climate change has led to increasing weather-related disasters. Population expansion and human encroachment on animals' natural habitats could potentially lead to further pandemic events. Expansion of military capabilities, including weapons of mass destruction, has the potential to cause large-scale casualties both in urban areas and on the battlefield. In all of these cases, our health care systems will require strong leadership and creative, adaptive physicians and staff to navigate unchartered waters. There is no physician better positioned to lead through these challenging times than an anesthesiologist.

Jesse Raiten, MD
Department of Anesthesiology and Critical Care
Perelman School of Medicine
of the University of Pennsylvania
3400 Spruce Street, Dulles 6
Philadelphia, PA 19104, USA

Lee A. Fleisher, MD, FACC, FAHA
Perelman School of Medicine
University of Pennsylvania
3400 Spruce Street, Dulles 680
Philadelphia, PA 19104, USA

E-mail addresses:
Jesse.Raiten@pennmedicine.upenn.edu (J. Raiten)
Lee.Fleisher@uphs.upenn.edu (L.A. Fleisher)

Development of an Anesthesiology Disaster Response Plan

Mac Staben, MD, MA, Jesse Raiten, MD*,
Meghan Lane-Fall, MD, MSHP, Michael Scott, MB ChB

KEYWORDS

- Disaster planning • Anesthesiology • Coronavirus • Earthquakes • Disasters
- COVID-19

KEY POINTS

- The COVID-19 pandemic has demonstrated the importance of thorough disaster planning for anesthesiologists.
- Work done in emergency medicine and prior experiences in disaster settings should inform disaster planning strategies for the future.
- Disasters put health care workers at risk for physical and emotional harm.

INTRODUCTION

The World Health Organization defines a disaster as "a serious disruption of the functioning of a community or a society causing widespread human, material, economic or environmental losses which exceed the ability of the affected community or society to cope using its own resources."[1] Disasters can have a profound effect on the demand for health care and its delivery, as seen across a variety of events, including Hurricane Katrina; earthquakes in Bam, Iran, and in Haiti; and the response to regional or global pandemics, such as the Ebola outbreak in western Africa from 2014 to 2016 as well as the ongoing COVID-19 pandemic. Effectively caring for patients at all times requires disaster preparation. In the United States alone, the year 2020 has seen a significant number of disasters, including the COVID-19 pandemic, wildfires across the western United States, and a large number of devastating hurricanes and storms across the southeastern United States, all contributing to significant loss of life and property.

Managing the aftermath of these events has required coordinated, strong responses from the health care industry. Because many disasters give no warning, successfully managing the health care implications of a disaster requires the preemptive

Department of Anesthesiology and Critical Care, Perelman School of Medicine of the University of Pennsylvania, 3400 Spruce Street, Dulles 6, Philadelphia, PA 19104, USA
* Corresponding author.
E-mail address: Jesse.Raiten@pennmedicine.upenn.edu

Anesthesiology Clin 39 (2021) 245–253
https://doi.org/10.1016/j.anclin.2021.02.001
1932-2275/21/© 2021 Elsevier Inc. All rights reserved.
anesthesiology.theclinics.com

development of a thorough, comprehensive strategy to effectively use health care personnel, facilities, and equipment. Whether it is an isolated event, such as a flood, or a prolonged affair, such as the COVID-19 pandemic, disasters frequently are dynamic, and response plans must be adaptable to rapidly changing circumstances. In the case of a health care crisis, these may include changes in staffing models, geographic patient locations, personal protective equipment, and numerous other elements.

This article discusses different types of disasters, including those that cause disruptions to physical structures and ones that do not. The specific roles of anesthesiologists during a disaster response and the various ways that anesthesiologists can contribute individually and in collaboration with other health care providers are considered. A robust literature for disaster planning from different specialties and government agencies already exists, so the contributions from other medical fields, including trauma surgery and emergency medicine, are reviewed. Disaster planning and several examples of disaster plans, which are documents and strategies that guide the acquisition of resources and allow health systems to execute adaptive and flexible plans once a disaster does occur, are discussed. Special attention is paid to the role of anesthesiologists in the creation and implementation of a disaster response plan. The effects that responding to a disaster can have on medical personnel also are considered. Disasters can have a direct impact on health care providers (physical injuries) or secondary impacts, such as through financial loss or psychological trauma. The various types of injuries, both physical and psychological, and their impact on health care workers, are considered.

DISCUSSION
Types of Disasters

There are many ways to classify disasters, but, in terms of their impact on health care, one way to distinguish them is by considering whether or not they have caused physical damage to health care facilities and the infrastructure that supports them. In cases of many mass casualty events, ranging from transportation accidents to mass shootings, the stress on the health care system comes from the need to triage patients and to effectively manage a surge in demand from injured patients. In response to these disasters, hospitals in the United States largely use the Hospital Incident Command System, which outlines a command structure and responsibilities in the response to a mass casualty incident (**Fig. 1**).[2] A major consideration in these types of mass casualty events involves adequate marshalling of resources and triaging of patients.

Events, such as earthquakes, hurricanes, and other natural disasters, may cause an even more challenging situation, whereby health care infrastructure and the physical hospital may be damaged, thereby limiting the actual ability of physicians and the health care team to actually provide care. For example, during the earthquake in Haiti in 2010, 8 hospitals were destroyed and 22 seriously damaged in the 3 regions most affected by the earthquake.[3] The destruction of these hospitals significantly limited their abilities to provide immediate care to patients. Similarly, following the fertilizer explosion in Beirut in 2020, several hospitals were destroyed or damaged, whereby they could not treat patients.

After a significant event, a damaged hospital may be unable to respond fully. Crucial supplies like water, oxygen, and electricity can be disrupted, as was the case where water supplies were disrupted at the main prefecture hospital following the Fukushima, Japan, earthquake in 2011. After that event roads were severely damaged, limiting the abilities of staff to commute to the hospital and transport patients or for

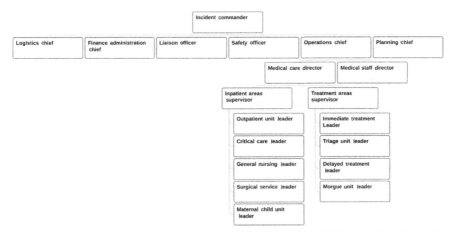

Fig. 1. Hospital incident command system. (*Modified from* Born CT, Briggs SM, Ciraulo DL, Frykberg ER, Hammond JS, et al. Disasters and Mass Casualties: I. General Principles of Response and Management, J Am Acad Orthop Surg, 2007.)

the health care system to move patients between facilities.[4] In the perioperative environment, critical resources like lighting, oxygen, and water often are taken for granted, but during a disaster these basic utilities can be disrupted, necessitating the transfer of patients to other facilities. Comprehensive disaster plans must anticipate these challenges and outline plans to mitigate the effects of loss of critical infrastructure and mechanisms to transfer patients to intact health care facilities when needed.

The Role of Anesthesiologists During a Disaster

Anesthesiologists are uniquely qualified to participate in a disaster response (**Fig. 2**). Research has shown that after an earthquake approximately half of all injuries involve fractures of some kind, many needing operative interventions.[5] Anesthesiologists have a variety of modalities for providing anesthesia, some of which are well-suited to disaster or limited-resource settings. Nevertheless, the anesthesia delivered under disaster conditions will likely vary significantly from the anesthetics typically provided under stable conditions.

Understanding the scope of anesthesia provided in low-income and middle-income countries helps illustrate the types of anesthesia that may be safely provided under disaster conditions. In a review of 467 hospitals in low-income and middle-income countries, only 50% had reliable electricity, defined as fewer than 2 outages per week. Only 61% of hospitals reported having a reliable oxygen source in the operating rooms, and 51% of hospitals had a functioning pulse oximeter. Similarly, the types of anesthetics delivered varied significantly from anesthesia typically provided in high-income countries. Ketamine was reported by 73% of hospitals as the most frequently used anesthetic because of its ability to preserve hemodynamic stability and allow patients to breathe spontaneously, without the need for supplementary oxygen.[6]

Similarly, in the setting of a disaster or an armed conflict, the types of anesthetics delivered vary significantly from those provided in stable, resource-rich environments. In a disaster setting, resources like oxygen and power may be unavailable. A review of Médecins Sans Frontières (MSF) anesthetics showed that in their response to the 2010 earthquake in Haiti, 66% of anesthetics were general (nonintubated), 21% were spinal, 4% other, and only 9% general anesthesia with endotracheal intubation. In MSF's response to the civil war in Syria, 48% of anesthetics were general

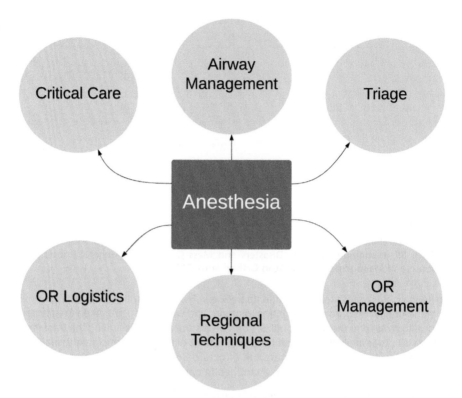

Fig. 2. Anesthesiologists are versatile members of a disaster response team and can participate in numerous clinical and leadership capacities. OR, operating room.

(nonintubated), 28% were spinal, and 18% were general anesthesia with endotracheal intubation.[7] This stands in marked contrast to many developed countries, for example, the United Kingdom, where the National Health Service report that 77% of their anesthetics were general (44.6% of patients received an endotracheal tube and 51.3% received a supraglottic airway device).[8] During a disaster, anesthesiologists most likely do not have the same equipment that is routinely available, and the anesthesia disaster response plan must reflect this. Stockpiles of drugs, such as ketamine and local anesthetics, more suited to providing anesthesia in disaster settings, should be maintained.

Regional anesthesia has many potential benefits in disaster or resource-limited settings, partially due to its ability to maintain a patient's spontaneous ventilation. Prior studies have demonstrated that regional anesthesia is a rapid and safe method for reducing pain caused by limb trauma. Therefore, it may have a role in improving pain management during the initial response to a major earthquake or other disaster where traumatic injuries are common. Unfortunately, no randomized studies exist examining the effectiveness, safety, or acceptability of regional anesthesia following a major earthquake.[9]

Anesthesiologists in a disaster setting can expect to be limited in terms of the drugs, resources, and logistical systems that they may be accustomed too, like oxygen or power, as discussed previously. Personnel shortages, however, such as not having enough anesthesiologists, may act as a bottleneck in the acute phase of a disaster response. This may be evident particularly in disasters with many associated traumatic injuries that require surgical and, therefore, anesthesia services.

Anesthesiologists' training is broad, and their skill sets are widely applicable. By virtue of their extensive training in resuscitation and management of critically ill patients, anesthesiologists are competent to perform many procedures and to manage patients requiring intensive care. As airway specialists, anesthesiologists can be called to assist in intubations, placement of supraglottic airways, or obtaining vascular access. In events requiring rapid patient triage, anesthesiologists can assess a patient's degrees of hemodynamic instability and need for urgent intervention. Anesthesiologists often manage patient flow through the perioperative setting and may continue to oversee patient placement and transition between the preoperative, intraoperative, and postoperative phases.

Anesthesiologists involved with disaster management should leverage the already abundant literature and resources available from other medical specialties. Emergency medicine providers, in particular, have published extensive literature about disaster response and triage. Currently, the American College of Emergency Physicians lists 23 dedicated fellowship programs in disaster medicine.[10] A multidisciplinary approach to disaster management planning is beneficial for all parties and may lead to more efficient and effective strategies for the hospital as a whole to approach a disaster.

In the case of COVID-19, the anesthesiologists' role during the pandemic included intraoperative as well as intensive care unit care, working in conjunction with practitioners from multiple medical specialties. A drop in surgical volume allowed anesthesia providers to be tasked to other jobs, such as critical care and respiratory therapy. Surgical volume fell during the pandemic across many specialties and may have created a backlog of cases for years to come. For example, a large number of spinal surgeries were delayed.[11]

Disaster Planning

Disasters are defined by the Federal Emergency Management Agency as having 4 phases: mitigation, preparedness, response, and recovery.[12] Mitigation involves attempting to diminish the possibility or severity of a problem before it begins. These efforts can exist either on a local level, such as ensuring that building codes are enforced and adequate to withstand natural disasters like earthquakes, or on a global scale, by advocating for decreased carbon emissions in order to reduce the risk of catastrophic wildfires or hurricanes.

Governmental organizations are likely to have a significant role in outlining mitigation efforts, but anesthesiologists always will be able to advocate for this kind of action. Preparedness involves planning, training, and educational activities to respond to events that cannot be mitigated. Such activities may include creating and maintaining a stockpile of important medications, developing phone trees and chains of command for eventual disasters, or simulations. Once a disaster occurs, the 2 following phases are response and recovery. The response phase begins immediately after the event and involves the active response to a disaster. The final phase is recovery. During recovery, restoration efforts occur simultaneously with regular, predisaster types of operations and activities. The recovery period from a disaster can be prolonged and can lead to significant stress for those suffering from and responding to a disaster. Additionally, during all of these phases, patients continue to need health care, so a health care system must be able to provide medical care while also dealing with the acute injuries to patients harmed by the disaster.

Since September 11, 2001, there has been keen interest in improving disaster planning. Some regulatory bodies require that hospitals maintain up-to-date disaster plans. There also have been increased regulatory requirements for hospitals and other health care facilities to develop their own disaster planning and carry out regular testing and drills. Significant work into disaster planning already has been accomplished throughout the medical field, and a wide variety of disaster plans are available as templates from different institutions. This can be seen within both societies for anesthesiology and other academic societies in medicine. For example, the American Society of Anesthesiologists provides a checklist for mass casualty events. The American College of Emergency Physicians has put forward a hospital checklist (originally created as a survey for hospitals) that discusses many of the useful elements for a disaster plan and includes concrete questions about the preparedness and facilities available that may be used in the event of a disaster. By completing this checklist, a facility may learn about its own disaster preparedness and potential areas for improvement.[13]

Disaster plans vary between hospitals based on projected patient volumes, types of patients, and available resources. One important aspect of disaster planning involves the shifting of personnel and materials between different hospitals or health care facilities. In a disaster, different facilities may be affected at different times. Although 1 hospital may be overwhelmed, capacity may exist within the health system as a whole. This applies not only to physical bed availability but also to drug and personnel resources. This was seen during the COVID-19 pandemic, as many hospitals reported shortages of essential drugs, such as propofol, midazolam, fentanyl, rocuronium, and cisatracurium—all critical medications in the anesthesia and intensive care environments.[14] Effective disaster planning requires a centralized system for assessing the supply needs of affected hospitals and redistributing resources as needed.

Disaster simulation can be a valuable tool in preparing for an actual event. A simulation held by the Italian Society of Anesthesia, Analgesia, Resuscitation and Intensive Care demonstrated that a multiday disaster simulation was deemed "an invaluable experience for the anesthesiology trainees, providing them with the skill set to understand the fundamental principles of a mass-casualty response."[15] Practically, simulation benefits participants by improving their abilities to manage disasters.[16] Simulation of responses to a mass casualty incident has been shown to improve the ability of practitioners to triage patients correctly.[17] By simulating disaster scenarios, hospitals will be able to perform more effectively and anticipate the potential difficulties in the event of a true calamity.

Preventing Harm to Health Care Workers

In responding to a disaster, health care workers may suffer physical or psychological harm. Disaster situations may create political instability where hospitals and health care facilities can either be targeted, as occurred in both Syria and Yemen, or fall victim to violence. A report by Physicians for Human Rights noted that during 2019, in countries where the organization worked, there were at least 1200 incidents of violence against health care workers, with at least 150 medical workers killed.[18] A concrete plan for ensuring the security of health care facilities should be a provision of any disaster plan.

The COVID-19 pandemic clearly has shown the risk health care workers assume when working in a disaster environment. As of October 19, 2020, according to the Centers for Disease Control and Prevention, more than 180,000 health care workers have been infected with the novel coronavirus, resulting in 757 deaths.[19] At the beginning of the pandemic, concern existed about supplies of personal protective equipment, with many hospitals requiring reuse of masks. Extensive research into methods for conserving, disinfecting, and reusing such equipment is ongoing. Health care workers are at increased risk of contracting COVID-19, in particular those with inadequate personal protective equipment.[20]

The danger posed to health care workers participating in disaster relief extends beyond the immediate risk to life and limb to more insidious psychological stressors. At baseline, health care workers are at an elevated risk of experiencing symptoms of anxiety, depression, or burnout. The prevalence of depression, or depressive symptoms, among resident physicians has been estimated to be as high as 28.8%.[21] Compared with working US adults, US physicians were more likely to have symptoms of burnout (37.9% vs 27.8%, respectively) and to be dissatisfied with work-life balance (40.2% vs 23.2%, respectively).[22] Physicians also have been shown to be at an increased risk of suicide compared with the general population.[23] Prior disasters have been shown to negatively affect the mental health of caregivers. A study comparing negative psychological outcomes among workers who took care of patients with severe acute respiratory syndrome (SARS) in Toronto, Canada, demonstrated significantly higher levels of burnout, psychological distress, and posttraumatic stress than their peers at hospitals that did not accept such patients.[24] It is clear that those who respond to a disaster are at elevated risk for developing significant problems, both psychological and physical.[25]

Similar issues have been seen in health care workers during the COVID-19 pandemic. A survey of health care workers in China during the early phases of the pandemic demonstrated high levels of depression, stress, anxiety, distress, anger, fear, insomnia, and posttraumatic stress disorder, with the greatest risk factor for distress being a frontline or emergency health care worker.[26,27] Although health care systems have faced similar types of challenges before, data suggest that the rates of distress among health care workers caring for patients with COVID-19 surpass those reported after Ebola, SARS, and other pandemics.[27]

Interventions exist to mitigate the negative impact on the mental health of people who are caring for patients during a pandemic.[28] A comprehensive disaster plan should include strategies to support providers who suffer from posttraumatic stress disorder or other psychological effects due to providing care for patients during times of disaster.

SUMMARY

An effective response to a disaster requires the preemptive creation and practice of a disaster response plan. Anesthesiologists are well suited to play a central role in the drafting and implementation of such plans, at both the hospital and regional levels. Disaster planning already is required by many health care systems, but by actively engaging with disaster response teams in the hospitals and focusing on ways to collaborate with other departments, anesthesiologists can have a positive impact on care and patient outcomes during critical times.

CLINICS CARE POINTS

- Anesthesiologists should collaborate with hospital leadership during times of crisis to enact disaster response plans and optimize patient care.
- Anesthesiologists should draw from existing work and expertise in emergency medicine, prior disaster responses, and published protocols when creating a disaster response plan.

- Health care workers responding to disasters are at high risk for physical and psychological trauma. Although evidence-based best practices do not yet exist, preventing and ameliorating this harm are crucial.
- When providing clinical care in a disaster setting, anesthesiologists should consider regional and spinal anesthesia, which facilitates spontaneous ventilation.

DISCLOSURE

The authors have nothing to disclose.

REFERENCES

1. Humanitarian Health Action. World Health Organization. Available at: https://www. who.int/hac/about/definitions/en/. Accessed November 9, 2020.
2. Born CT, Briggs SM, Ciraulo DL, et al. Disasters and Mass Casualties: I. General Principles of Response and Management. J Am Acad Orthop Surg 2007;15(7): 388–96.
3. PanAmerican Health Organization. Earthquake in Haiti. Available at: https://www. paho.org/disasters/index.php?option=com_content&view=article&id=1088:the-latest-from-haiti&Itemid=906&lang=en#:~:text=Eight%20hospitals%20were% 20totally%20destroyed,Nippes%2C%20Sud%2DEst). Accessed November 9, 2020.
4. Murakawa M. Anesthesia department preparedness for a multiple-casualty incident: lessons learned from the Fukushima earthquake and the Japanese nuclear power disaster. Anesthesiol Clin 2013;31(1):117–25.
5. Lu-Ping Z, Rodriguez-Llanes JM, Qi W, et al. Multiple injuries after earthquakes: a retrospective analysis on 1,871 injured patients from the 2008 Wenchuan earthquake. Crit Care 2012;16(3):R87.
6. Dohlman Lena. Providing anesthesia in resource-limited settings. Curr Opin Anaesthesiol 2017;30(4):496–500.
7. Trelles Centurion M, Van Den Bergh R, Gray H. Anesthesia provision in disasters and armed conflicts. Curr Anesthesiol Rep 2017;7(1):1–7.
8. Sury MR, Palmer JH, Cook TM, et al. The State of UK anaesthesia: a survey of National Health Service activity in 2013. Br J Anaesth 2014;113(4):575–84.
9. Aluisio AR, Teicher C, Wiskel T, et al. Focused Training for Humanitarian Responders in Regional Anesthesia Techniques for a Planned Randomized Controlled Trial in a Disaster Setting. PLoS Curr 2016;8. https://doi.org/10.1371/ currents.dis.e75f9f9d977ac8adededb381e3948a04.
10. American College of Emergency Physicians: Disaster Medicine Fellowships. Available at: https://www.acep.org/how-we-serve/sections/disaster-medicine/ disaster-medicine-fellowships/. Accessed November 10, 2020.
11. Jain A, Jain P, Aggarwal S. SARS-CoV-2 impact on elective orthopaedic surgery: implications for post- pandemic recovery. J Bone Joint Surg Am 2020;102(13):e68.
12. Emergency Management in the United States. Available at: https://training.fema. gov/emiweb/downloads/is111_unit%204.pdf. Accessed November 10, 2020.
13. Hospital Disaster Preparedness Self-Assessment Tool. Emergency Preparedness. Available at: https://www.calhospitalprepare.org/post/hospital-disaster-preparedness-self-assessment-tool. Accessed November 10, 2020.
14. Shuman AG, Fox ER, Unguru Y. COVID-19 and drug shortages: a call to action. J Manag Care Spec Pharm 2020;26(8):945–7.

15. Carenzo L, Bazurro S, Colombo D, et al. An Island-wide disaster drill to train the next generation of anesthesiologists: The SIAARTI Academy Experience. Disaster Med Public Health Prep 2020;2:1–4.
16. Bartley BH, Stella JB, Walsh LD. What a disaster?! Assessing utility of simulated disaster exercise and educational process for improving hospital preparedness. Prehosp Disaster Med 2006;21(4):249–55.
17. Cicero MX, Auerbach MA, Zigmont J, et al. Simulation training with structured debriefing improves residents' pediatric disaster triage performance. Prehosp Disaster Med 2012;27(3):239–44.
18. Health Workers at Risk: Violence Against Health Care. Available at: https://www.safeguardinghealth.org/sites/shcc/files/SHCC2020final.pdf. Accessed November 10, 2020.
19. CDC Covid Data Tracker. Centers for Disease Control and Prevention. Available at: https://covid.cdc.gov/covid-data-tracker/?CDC_AA_refVal=https%3A%2F%2Fwww.cdc.gov%2Fcoronavirus%2F2019-ncov%2Fcases-updates%2Fcases-in-us.html#health-care-personnel. Accessed November 10, 2020.
20. Nguyen LH, Drew DA, Graham MS, et al. Risk of COVID-19 among front-line health-care workers and the general community: a prospective cohort study. Lancet Public Health 2020;5(9):e475–83.
21. Mata DA, Ramos MA, Bansal N, et al. Prevalence of depression and depressive symptoms among resident physicians: a systematic review and meta-analysis. JAMA 2015;314(22):2373–83.
22. Shanafelt TD, Boone S, Tan L, et al. Burnout and Satisfaction With Work-Life Balance Among US Physicians Relative to the General US Population. Arch Intern Med 2012;172(18):1377–85.
23. Dutheil F, Aubert C, Pereira B, et al. Suicide among physicians and health-care workers: A systematic review and meta-analysis. PLoS One 2019;14(12):e0226361.
24. Maunder RG, Lancee WJ, Balderson KE, et al. Long-term psychological and occupational effects of providing hospital healthcare during SARS outbreak. Emerg Infect Dis 2006;12(12):1924–32.
25. Garbern SC, Ebbeling LG, Bartels SA. A Systematic Review of Health Outcomes Among Disaster and Humanitarian Responders. Prehosp Disaster Med 2016; 31(6):635–42.
26. Shaukat N, Ali DM, Razzak J. Physical and mental health impacts of COVID-19 on healthcare workers: a scoping review. Int J Emerg Med 2020;13(1):40.
27. Lai J, Ma S, Wang Y, et al. Factors associated with mental health outcomes among health care workers exposed to coronavirus disease 2019. JAMA Netw Open 2020;3(3):e203976.
28. Shultz JM, Baingana F, Neria Y. The 2014 Ebola outbreak and mental health: current status and recommended response. JAMA 2015;313(6):567–8.

The Initial Response to a Pandemic: Anesthesiology Experiences from China at the Onset of COVID-19

Jing Wu, MD, PhD[a], Xueyin Chen, MD[a], Xiangdong Chen, MD, PhD[a],
Shanglong Yao, MD, PhD[a],*, Renyu Liu, MD, PhD[b],*

KEYWORDS

- Anesthesia • Perioperative management • COVID-19 • Infection control

KEY POINTS

- Education, training, and constant update of coronavirus disease 2019 (COVID-19)–related knowledge and skills are vital during the pandemic.
- A well-designed and effective response system during the outbreak of COVID-19 is crucial for the safety of both patients and health care providers.
- In extreme situations such as the COVID-19 pandemic, anesthesiologists may transform into internists, while continuing to use their specialty skills in airway management and mechanical ventilation.
- During the pandemic, anesthesiologists acquired skills in personal protective equipment, infectious disease, and management of patients outside of the operating rooms.

INTRODUCTION

Since December 2019, a total of 41 cases of pneumonia of unknown cause, which were later identified from a novel virus named SARS-CoV-2 (severe acute respiratory syndrome coronavirus 2), have been confirmed in Wuhan city, Hubei Province, China.[1,2] The disease was officially named coronavirus disease 2019 (COVID-19) by the World Health Organization (WHO). On January 30, the WHO Emergency Committee declared the 2019 novel coronavirus outbreak a public health emergency of international concern (PHEIC).[3] With a population of more than 12 million people,

[a] Department of Anesthesiology, Institute of Anesthesia and Critical Care Medicine, Union Hospital, Tongji Medical College, Huazhong University of Science and Technology, 1277 Jiefang Avenue, Wuhan, Hubei 430022, China; [b] Department of Anesthesiology and Critical Care, Perelman School of Medicine at the University of Pennsylvania, Center of Penn Global Health Scholar, 336 John Morgan Building, 3620 Hamilton Walk, Philadelphia, PA 19104, USA
* Corresponding authors.
E-mail addresses: ysltian@163.com (S.Y.); RenYu.Liu@pennmedicine.upenn.edu (R.L.)

Anesthesiology Clin 39 (2021) 255–264
https://doi.org/10.1016/j.anclin.2021.02.002
1932-2275/21/© 2021 Elsevier Inc. All rights reserved.

Wuhan was the first city, and also the hardest-hit city, in China forced to deal with the outbreak of COVID-19. Since February 11, 2020, after being assigned as the designated hospital, Union Hospital, one of the biggest general hospitals in Wuhan, had reconstructed 3 districts specifically for treating a total of 5200 patients with COVID-19, mainly patients with severe or critical disease. At the same time, the hospital also managed 2 temporary COVID-19 specialty hospitals (named Fangchang Hospitals), providing treatment of more than 200,00 asymptomatic or mildly symptomatic patients with COVID-19.

The limited information about the virus increased the difficulty of predicting the required medical resources, and challenged almost all subspecialties of medicine. Anesthesiologists are not traditionally infection control professionals. Because of strict rules of aseptic technique in the operating room (OR), anesthesiologists are traditionally good at prevention and control of nosocomial infection during the perioperative period, resulting in a more positive attitude to fight against the epidemic. Meanwhile, expertise in resuscitation and basic life support makes anesthesiologists more active in participating in the treatment of severe and critical patients with COVID-19 in the multidisciplinary intensive care setting.

This article documents experiences of frontline anesthesia providers in Wuhan, mainly from the anesthesiologists in Union Hospital, Tongji Medical College, Huazhong University of Science and Technology, Wuhan, Hubei, China. It is hoped that these experiences can document valuable processes used to optimize the emergency response system, the arrangement of medical resources and emergency allocation, as well as provide insight into anesthesiologists' roles in expanding their practices and driving innovation to improve patient care.

TIME PERIODS CLASSIFIED BY KEY EVENTS AND INTERVENTION

Key events and interventions are helpful to understand the dynamics of the COVID-19 outbreak in Wuhan. One key event is Chunyun (massive human movement because of the Chinese New Year festival) from January 10 to 22. The other key event is large-scale city lockdowns in China, including Wuhan, from January 23 to March 8. A report about the COVID-19 outbreak in Wuhan classified the epidemiology of this epidemic into 5 periods: December 8 to January 9 (no intervention), January 10 to 22 (Chunyun), January 23 to February 1 (cordons sanitaire, traffic restriction, and home quarantine), February 2 to 16 (centralized quarantine and treatment), and February 17 to March 8 (universal symptom survey).[4] In addition to these key events and associated epidemiologic features, several suspected cases at the early stage, and related nosocomial transmission, also had an impact on medical responses to the pandemic. Accordingly, the initial response can also be classified into 2 time periods: an early-warning period from January 10 to 18, and a full-scale-launch period in the whole hospital after January 19.

Early Warnings

Our early warning came from a specific patient treated in our hospital during the perioperative period before the outbreak of COVID-19. This patient is a milestone in the recognition of human-to-human transmission, before clinicians really paid attention to this pneumonia of unknown cause. A 70-year-old male patient was admitted in late December, 2019, and was scheduled for intranasal endoscopic surgery. Because of his past medical history of hypertension, diabetes, and heart attack, preoperative consultation and anesthesia evaluation were performed twice, on December 31, 2019 and January 3, 2020. The surgery was performed under total intravenous anesthesia in a regular OR on January 6, 2020. After a 2-hour operation, he was transferred to the postanesthesia care unit and was extubated peacefully. He was transferred to the neurosurgery ward 30 minutes later. The patient developed a fever 3 days after surgery and was diagnosed with pneumonia of unknown cause. On January 18, 12 days after his operation, his oral swab tested positive for SARS-CoV-2. He was immediately transferred to an isolation ward for 1 week before being transferred to one of the first-batch designated hospitals in Wuhan. He died of respiratory failure 4 weeks after surgery.

Because the patient had no epidemiologic history and clinical manifestations related to COVID-19 before surgery, no COVID-19 investigation was performed then, and the medical staff only used standard protection during the perioperative diagnosis and treatment periods. Four nurses in the neurosurgery ward, who had direct contact with him before quarantine without protective equipment, were infected, and 10 more staff in the ward who did not contact him directly later tested positive.[5] None of the anesthesia providers tested positive.

After January 10, when the patient was diagnosed with pneumonia of unknown cause, terminal disinfection of the anesthesia machine was immediately performed, and the follow-up patients in the same OR were traced. None of the patients developed a related infection. Later, the terminal disinfection of the anesthesia machine expanded to all of the neurosurgery ORs. Meanwhile, personal protective equipment (PPE) was increased throughout perioperative neuroanesthesia care, by wearing double gloves, double surgical masks, and disposable operating clothes as outer layers. At the same time, the hospital started an early detection and reporting system of suspected cases. Since then, our department has started to use PPE in every emergency surgery unit.

Full-Scale Launch

On January 18, an emergency meeting was held to review the epidemic situation of COVID-19 and emphasize that infection control was the top priority. Temporary notices and training rules regarding infection prevention and control were released throughout the hospital, including different levels of recommended protection based on risk, and paying special attention to the potential for virus transmission via the aerosolized route.

On January 19 and 20, information focusing on perioperative infection control was released to the department staff, referencing WHO and Centers for Disease Control and Prevention (CDC) guidelines. It included precautions for infection control in the perioperative setting, personnel emergency allocation workflow, and tracking and management of medical staff after suspected and confirmed exposures to patients with COVID-19.

SYSTEM: ANESTHESIA AND INFECTION CONTROL MANAGEMENT

Based within the division of the Anesthesia Quality Control Team in the Department of Anesthesiology, an emergency infection control team was established. A total of 12 members were assigned to different divisions, including infection control training and supervision, education and training, daily routine disinfection processes, and resource and PPE management.

Workflow of Perioperative Infection Control

The emergency infection control team formulated the following workflow covering perioperative infection control in and out of the OR, to ensure the quality and safety of clinical anesthesia providers and patients, and prevent nosocomial infection:

1. Triage of suspected or confirmed cases of novel coronavirus pneumonia before entering the OR
2. Anesthetic checklist for suspected or confirmed cases of novel coronavirus pneumonia in the OR
3. Checklist of monitoring anesthesia care outside the OR during the outbreak of COVID-19, including sedation and anesthesia for gastrointestinal endoscopic and fiberoptic bronchoscopic procedures
4. Requirements for disinfection and sterilization of the environment, surfaces, instruments, and equipment in the OR during the outbreak of COVID-19
5. Personal protection requirements for medical staff in the OR
6. Personal protection requirements for anesthesiologists when performing emergency endotracheal intubation in the fever clinic or isolation ward
7. Infection control anesthetic requirements for anesthetic evaluation in the Preoperative Evaluation Center

Infection control precautions in the perioperative setting involve at least 3 stages: preoperative triage, infection control management intraoperatively, and infection control during postoperative patient transport. There was a high degree of familiarity with procedures in the OR setting already, so greater attention was paid to infection control management outside the OR at the early stage of the outbreak, such as in outpatient services, emergency endotracheal intubation in the fever clinic or isolation ward, and preanesthetic evaluation area. In general, it was easier to maintain high vigilance and strictly follow the safety protocols in clinical workplaces; however, non–work-related contact between medical staff generated a higher exposure risk, such as when dining together, because all medical staff may have been infected. Therefore, posting the key points of infection control in both the clinical and nonclinical settings, and maintaining a high level of vigilance and sterility, was important toward mitigating disease transmission.

Education, Training, and Updating

Education, training, and constant updates of COVID-19–related knowledge and skills are vital during the pandemic. Maintaining appropriate education includes the review of guidelines issued by the National Health Commission in China and the WHO, and protocols developed by the hospital. In order to avoid staff gathering, face-to-face and simulation instruction were replaced by online learning, including text materials and PowerPoint presentations, and instructional videos. Video conference also played an important role, allowing real-time discussion and feedback. During the training, it is particularly important to practice the standard process of donning and doffing of PPE. Formal information-sharing channels for medical staff should be encouraged through professional networks and diversified social media. Since June 2020, the National Conference on Medical Education has offered nationwide educational opportunities discussing various aspects of COVID-19, such as training on nucleic acid testing and epidemiologic investigation, which are mandatory requirements for all medical staff in China, and these are free for 1 year (http://www.ncme.org.cn).

STAFF: NEW WORK MODEL AND ALLOCATION OF ANESTHESIOLOGISTS

The COVID-19 pandemic challenged health systems and providers, and disrupted medical care. As the epidemic progressed, the work of our anesthesiologists progressed out of the OR setting and into a more multidisciplinary team model of epidemic prevention and control, requiring anesthesiologists to work in a variety of locations. Anesthesiologists were not unique in the expansion of their clinical roles, because physicians from other medical specialties also returned to general medical practice. The balance of allocation of anesthesiologists between clinical anesthesia and COVID-19–related care needed continuous adjustments throughout the pandemic.

Clinical Work

Before experiencing an unprecedented surge of COVID-19 cases, clinical anesthesia was still our routine work mode. As indicated in **Fig. 1**, the number of monthly anesthesia cases in Union Hospital decreased from 8194 in December, 2019, to 5277 in January, 2020, in which emergency anesthesia comprised 1151 and 632 respectively.

Because epidemic control was considered the top priority, prompt risk assessment and strict measures to limit infection spread within the hospital, and to health care workers, were strictly enforced. The concept of flattening the curve by delaying the peak of the epidemic, aimed to put less strain on health care capacity and reduce the medical burden on hospitals. As a result, most elective operations were canceled or postponed, so the number of monthly anesthesia cases decreased dramatically to 155 and 332 in February and April 2020, respectively. Concurrently, almost all clinical doctors from various specialties converted to infectious diseases doctors, or critical care physicians.

Epidemic Prevention and Control

On January 19, an emergency personnel staffing model for PHEIC was established on a voluntary basis, and included 2 anesthesiologists on standby (24 h/d) in case of public emergency. It was touching that the 28-doctor roster was soon filled by our courageous colleagues, covering the following 2 weeks, including Spring Festival. Since January 23, anesthesiologists were included in the hospital multidisciplinary medical team, including the fever clinic, observation room of the emergency department, and isolation wards in Union Hospital, as well as other designated hospitals in Wuhan. From January to April, a total of 48 anesthesiologists and 27 anesthesia nurses were allocated to the frontline, including 5 professors or associate professors, 14 attending doctors, 21 residents, and 8 interns.

Daily Reports and Tracking Possible Infections

Core principles of epidemic control, including early detection, early reporting, early isolation, early diagnosis, early treatment, and early control, were identified when

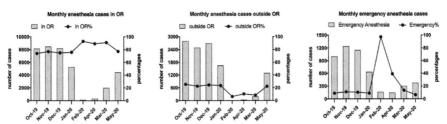

Fig. 1. Monthly anesthesia cases in the OR and outside the OR, and monthly emergency anesthesia cases. (*A*) Monthly anesthesia cases in OR: in OR% = (anesthesia cases in OR/total anesthesia cases) × 100%. (*B*) Monthly anesthesia cases outside OR: outside OR% = (anesthesia cases outside OR/total anesthesia cases) × 100%. (*C*) Monthly emergency anesthesia cases: emergency% = (emergency anesthesia cases/total anesthesia cases) × 100%. (*Data from* Union Hospital from October 2019 to May 2020.)

the epidemic began. A daily reporting system for all medical staff was initiated in February, 2020. All medical staff working in the hospital completed personal reporting every day via the hospital Web site, or mobile app (Wechat Official Account). Departmental reporting was important for tracking and management of medical staff who had potential or confirmed exposures. In the event of a medical staff (or cohabitating family) potential exposure, they were advised to quarantine for at least 2 weeks. For potential exposures, staff were evaluated to meet the following criteria:

1. An exposure history 2 weeks before onset: a history of direct or indirect contact to Wuhan-related seafood markets, or exposure to suspected or confirmed patients with COVID-19
2. Clinical manifestations: fever, cough, soreness, imaging features of viral pneumonia, normal or decreased leukocyte count, no significant improvement or progressive worsening after at least 3 days of regular antibiotic treatment

Because all staff worked in Wuhan, the epicenter of the pandemic, they were considered high risk for COVID-19 as long as they showed any related clinical manifestations. During the 2 -week observation, the body temperature and respiratory status were monitored every day and recorded. One member of our emergency infection control team closely tracked and conducted follow-up by daily telephone communication, or instant messaging. Further evaluations, such as nasopharyngeal swab examination for nucleic acid, blood test, C-reactive protein, and pulmonary imaging, were considered depending on the severity and progress of the patient's clinical symptoms. Our department had 4 anesthesiologists who contracted COVID-19; 3 of them were admitted and 1 received home quarantine before all of them fully recovered and returned to work.

RESOURCE MANAGEMENT
Epidemic Prevention Materials and Personal Protective Equipment Management

Resource management should be established as fast as possible because of the ongoing imbalance between supply and clinical demands. Because of the extended closure of factories, city lockdown, and the 14-day-long vacation of Chinese New Year, the supply of disposable items faced a state of persistent shortage at the early stage of the pandemic. It was a relief that almost all of the elective surgery was canceled or delayed, and the stock of supplies at last could support the requirements of emergent surgery. However, PPE had been badly needed since the beginning of the outbreak, so it was strictly managed and used according to different levels of precaution requirement. PPE, including disposable protective clothing, goggles, face screens, and N95 masks, was classified, counted, and checked by special personnel every day to ensure adequate supply for clinical service. In addition, unprecedented social measures, such as lockdowns, transport restrictions, and even food provision, came as new challenges to health providers. The hospital arranged accommodation and commuting for the frontline staff, as well as basic food provision for the staff working in the hospital. In addition, the department arranged for the nonfrontline clinical staff to provide services for care not related to COVID-19; in particular, emergency surgery.

Instruments and Equipment

Routine maintenance, cleaning, and disinfection of instruments and equipment was performed by special personnel. The authors noted that the malfunction rate of the anesthesia machine increased significantly after undergoing the frequent disinfection processes, thereby making the preoperative machine check particularly important. In the case of an unexpected machine failure, there should always be at least 1 additional anesthesia machine immediately available. In non–patient-care settings, ultraviolet lamp irradiation, plasma air disinfector, and chlorine-based disinfectant were used on a regular basis.

EXPERIENCE AND ACHIEVEMENTS
What Can Anesthesiologists Do on the Front Lines?

Considering the high risk of potential exposure to respiratory droplets or aerosol from patients' airways, the frontline anesthesiologists set up a 16-member team in charge of out-of-OR airway management throughout the hospital. The team was on call for 24 hours, and later expanded to provide sedation and analgesia, invasive respiratory and circulatory monitoring (eg, central venous catheterization, artery cannulation, and blood gas analysis), and cardiopulmonary ultrasonography examination for patients in isolation wards.

Because of changing clinical needs during the pandemic, the doctors in the isolation ward or intensive care unit (ICU) were composed of intensive care doctors and other specialists functioning as multidisciplinary teams. The setting up of an emergency team was a successful and rewarding experience, allowing anesthesiologists to focus on airway management and basic life support, areas in which they are experts. It also alleviated the pressure and exposure risk of the doctor in charge in the isolation wards. On account of the participation of anesthesiologists, the management of sedation and muscle relaxants for invasive mechanical ventilation, as well as the management of drug withdrawal and weaning from ventilator, was more standardized. In addition, anesthesiologists also provided resuscitation and supportive treatment under the guide of invasive monitoring and ultrasonography examination.

Since February 2020, more than 30 anesthesiologists were allocated to 8 isolation ICUs in the hospital, who participated in the treatment of more than 800 patients with COVID-19, including more than 300 severe and critical cases. The experience of perioperative management and emergency tracheal intubation of patients infected with COVID-19 has been summarized and presented in several publications.[6–9]

What Can Anesthesiologists Learn from the Front Lines?

Participating in the treatment of patients with COVID-19 improved the anesthesiologists' airway skills, in particular for patients with respiratory infections, as well as expanding knowledge of respiratory drugs (eg, aminophylline, glucocorticoids) and multiple means of oxygen therapy and ventilation. Our experience treating patients with COVID-19 also improved anesthesiologists' comfort and knowledge for the continuous management of critically ill patients. Participating in the whole process of COVID-19 treatment means that clinicians should not only focus on the temporary improvement but also consider the whole course and long-term prognosis for the patients. Anesthesiologists are used to focusing on patients' short-term treatment and outcome. For example, critically ill patients would be sent to the ICU after surgery, and transferred out of the ICU after extubation and achieving hemodynamic stability. During the treatment of COVID-19 in isolation wards, anesthesiologists, as well as other physicians, need to pay close attention to changes in patients' conditions, and make appropriate triage decisions. The multidisciplinary teams that worked in the isolation wards allowed physicians from different specialties to work together in patient care, with each providing their own areas of expertise and sharing their knowledge with other team members. This model of care was important to provide a constant high level of care, in the setting of understaffing and burnout seen during the pandemic.

The Response of Anesthesiology Societies in China: Chinese Association of Anesthesiologists and Chinese Society of Anesthesiology Task Force

In the early phase of the outbreak, the Chinese Society of Anesthesiology (CSA) and the Chinese Association of Anesthesiologists (CAA) jointly formed a task force and quickly drafted recommendations concerning the perioperative management of patients infected with the novel coronavirus.[7] These recommendations from the experts on the front lines aimed to provide suggestions on how to manage patients with COVID-19 in both the perioperative setting and in airway management for patients outside the OR. Moreover, CSA and CAA jointly set up the COVID-19 Prevention and Control Online Platform for Anesthesiologists on the official Web sites of both societies, with the goal to answer questions from anesthesiologists all over the country. According to incomplete statistics, more than 800 Chinese anesthesiologists and anesthetic nurses participated in the frontline medical work in Hubei Province. To provide assistance to providers experiencing psychological issues related to the pandemic, CAA and CSA also established a platform to provide free mental health care to all anesthesiologists and anesthetic nurses caring for patients with COVID-19. In addition, both associations held several online experience-sharing meetings with official anesthetic associations/societies around the world to share their firsthand experiences.

Research During the Pandemic

The pandemic presented an unprecedented challenge to rapidly develop new diagnostic, preventive, and therapeutic strategies. From the beginning of the pandemic, we collected and reported anesthesia-related clinical characteristics, as well as clinical outcomes of patients with confirmed or suspected COVID-19, and drafted protocols and procedures for anesthetic and airway management, as well as for infection control in the preanesthesia and OR settings.[9–11] Tracheal intubation in patients with COVID-19 was often necessary but had intrinsic danger to the anesthesiologist performing the procedure because of the potential for exposure to secretions and aerosols. The Chinese experience and guidelines for emergency endotracheal intubation in critically ill patients with COVID-19 were summarized, which helped keep health care workers safe and provide optimal airway management.[6,8]

The health of pregnant women, newborns, and children has also attracted much attention during the pandemic. Soon after COVID-19 presented, a case of successful spinal anesthesia was reported in a woman with confirmed COVID-19 undergoing emergency cesarean section, and a case of successful combined spinal and epidural anesthesia during an emergent cesarean delivery.[12,13] Moreover, the effects of underlying cardiovascular diseases on patients with COVID-19 have also been explored, as well as the damage caused by SARS-CoV-2 infection to the cardiovascular system.[14] It has been found that SARS-CoV-2 infection may damage the cardiovascular system, manifested as changes in cardiac structure and function, especially in the left heart and ascending aorta. In addition, anesthetic nurses also played key roles in caring for patients with COVID-19 in Fangchang Hospital, in the isolation wards, or in the ICU for critical cases. Results of the research conducted by anesthetic nurses showed that they can quickly adapt to the treatment and management of patients with COVID-19 because of their proficient skills in airway and respiratory management, as well as their rich experience in emergency responses and the use of life support equipment.[15]

Contribution to Guidelines

Consensus from experts who managed patients with COVID-19 could provide information in a more direct, structured, efficient, and reproducible way. Since the onset of COVID-19, the authors have drafted and published a series of professional recommendations and expert consensus statements concerning infection prevention and control in the Department of Anesthesiology, lessons learned and international expert recommendations on emergency tracheal intubation, and anesthetic management of special patient populations (elderly, maternal, and pediatric). As the medical order gradually returned to normal, the authors drafted the work recommendations for perioperative management during the recovery period following the pandemic. This series of expert recommendations and consensuses could help health care providers, particularly anesthesiologists, optimize the care of patients, the safety of their colleagues, and the public.

SUMMARY

Based on our experiences during the COVID-19 pandemic, the authors established protocols, guidelines, and a response system to effectively provide care to patients, while keeping ourselves safe from infection. With the pandemic ongoing, the so-called new normal in our practice will be based on ongoing training and education for staff, the ability to rapidly deploy health care providers when needed, and effective resource management. Because the future of the COVID-19 pandemic remains uncertain, constant updating and sharing of information will foster better care for patients, and a safer work environment for clinicians.

CLINICS CARE POINTS

- An emergency response system, that includes a new work model with proper allocation of manpower and medical resources, should be implemented as soon as possible when a disaster occurs.
- The protection of medical providers and patients are equally critical for a contagious deadly disease like COVID-19.
- Cancel or delay surgery when a deadly contagious disease with unknown etiology is suspected.

DISCLOSURE

The authors have nothing to disclose.

REFERENCES

1. Lu H, Stratton CW, Tang Y-W. Outbreak of pneumonia of unknown etiology in Wuhan, China: the mystery and the miracle. J Med Virol 2020;92:401–2.
2. WHO. Pneumonia of unknown cause – China. Available at: https://www.who.int/csr/don/05-january-2020-pneumonia-of-unkown-cause-china/en/.   Accessed February 25, 2021.
3. WHO. Clinical management of severe acute respiratory infection when novel coronavirus (nCoV) infection is suspected. Available at: https://www.who.int/publications-detail/clinical-management-of-severe-acute-respiratory-infectionwhen-novel-coronavirus-(ncov)-infection-is-suspected. Accessed February 25, 2021.
4. Pan A, Liu L, Wang C, et al. Association of public health interventions with the epidemiology of the COVID-19 outbreak in Wuhan, China. JAMA 2020;323:1–9.

5. Zhu W, Huang X, Zhao H, et al. A COVID-19 patient who underwent endonasal endoscopic pituitary adenoma resection: a case report. Neurosurgery 2020;87: E140–6.

6. Yao W, Wang T, Jiang B, et al. Emergency tracheal intubation in 202 patients with COVID-19 in Wuhan, China: lessons learnt and international expert recommendations. Br J Anaesth 2020;125:e28–37.

7. Chen X, Liu Y, Gong Y, et al. Perioperative management of patients infected with the novel coronavirus: recommendation from the joint task force of the Chinese Society of Anesthesiology and the Chinese Association of Anesthesiologists. Anesthesiology 2020;132(6):1307–16.

8. Xia H, Huang S, Xiao W, et al. Practical workflow recommendations for emergency endotracheal intubation in critically ill patients with COVID-19 based on the experience of Wuhan Union Hospital. J Clin Anesth 2020;66:109940.

9. Zhao S, Ling K, Yan H, et al. Anesthetic management of patients with COVID 19 infections during emergency procedures. J Cardiothorac Vasc Anesth 2020;34: 1125–31.

10. Xiangdong C, You S, Shanglong Y, et al. Perioperative care provider's considerations in managing patients with the COVID-19 infections. Transl Perioper Pain Med 2020;7(2):216–24.

11. Zhang H-F, Bo L, Lin Y, et al. Response of Chinese anesthesiologists to the COVID-19 outbreak. Anesthesiology 2020;132:1333–8.

12. Xia H, Zhao S, Wu Z, et al. Emergency Caesarean delivery in a patient with confirmed COVID-19 under spinal anaesthesia. Br J Anaesth 2020;124:e216–8.

13. Limin S, Weimin X, Ken L, et al. Anesthetic management for emergent cesarean delivery in a parturient with recent diagnosis of Coronavirus Disease 2019 (COVID-19): a case report. Transl Perioper Pain Med 2020;7:5–8.

14. Song L, Zhao S, Wang L, et al. Cardiovascular changes in patients with COVID-19 from Wuhan , China. Front Cardiovasc Med 2020;7:150.

15. Chen Q, Lan X, Zhao Z, Yao S. Role of anesthesia nurses in the treatment and management of patients with COVID-19. J Perianesth Nurs 2020;35(5):453–6.

Development of a Critical Care Response - Experiences from Italy During the Coronavirus Disease 2019 Pandemic

Emanuele Rezoagli, MD, PhD[a,b,*], Aurora Magliocca, MD, PhD[a],
Giacomo Bellani, MD, PhD[a,b], Antonio Pesenti, MD[c,d],
Giacomo Grasselli, MD[c,d]

KEYWORDS

- Critical care • Pandemic • Coronavirus disease 19 • COVID19 Lombardy Network
- Organizational response • Helmet continuous positive airway pressure
- Awake proning

KEY POINTS

- Italy was the first western country to face a large coronavirus disease 2019 (COVID-19) outbreak.
- COVID19 Lombardy Network responded to the surge of hospital admissions in Northern Italy; it organized a rapid increase in intensive care unit (ICU) beds and implemented measures for containment.
- Scientific evidence was provided by Italian centers to characterize the clinical history of COVID-19 associated respiratory failure.
- Relevant experience was collected in Italy during the pandemic about the use of noninvasive continuous positive airway pressure and awake proning, which were implemented to manage respiratory failure out of the ICU setting.
- Recommendations from national guidelines were structured to guide health care providers on resource allocation; promotion of awareness among Italian citizens within specific humanitarian and educational programs was implemented.

Funded by: CRUI2020.
[a] Department of Medicine and Surgery, University of Milano-Bicocca, Via Cadore, 48, Monza 20900, Italy; [b] Department of Emergency and Intensive Care, San Gerardo Hospital, Via G. B. Pergolesi, 33, Monza 20900, Italy; [c] Department of Pathophysiology and Transplantation, University of Milan, Via Francesco Sforza 35, Milano 20122, Italy; [d] Department of Anesthesia, Intensive Care and Emergency, Fondazione IRCCS Ca' Granda Ospedale Maggiore Policlinico, Via della Commenda, 10, Milano 20122, Italy
* Corresponding author. Department of Medicine and Surgery, University of Milano-Bicocca, Via Cadore 48, Monza (MB) 20900, Italy.
E-mail address: emanuele.rezoagli@unimib.it

Anesthesiology Clin 39 (2021) 265–284
https://doi.org/10.1016/j.anclin.2021.02.003
1932-2275/21/© 2021 Elsevier Inc. All rights reserved.

anesthesiology.theclinics.com

INTRODUCTION

Italy was the first western country facing an outbreak of coronavirus disease 2019 (COVID-19).[1] The first Italian patient diagnosed with COVID-19 was admitted, on Feb. 20, 2020, to the intensive care unit (ICU) in Codogno Hospital (Lodi, Lombardy, Italy), and the number of reported positive cases increased to 36 in the next 24 hours, and then exponentially for 18 days. This triggered a prompt, coordinated response of the ICUs in the epicenter region of the outbreak that resulted in a massive surge in the ICU bed capacity.[2]

An Italian registry from 3 northern Italian regions (Lombardy, Emilia-Romagna and Veneto) showed that the rate of ICU admission was 12.6% of COVID-19 hospital admissions. Eight hundred and five patients were admitted and treated in the ICU among 6378 patients hospitalized for COVID-19 in the period between Feb. 24 through March 8, 2020.[3] The coordination of a critical care response in Italy happened in collaboration with out-of-hospital, and out-of-ICU management of patients with respiratory failure.

Furthermore, as part of the implementation of an organizational response to the SARS-CoV2 outbreak, many Italian research groups collected data and provided scientific evidence to understand how to better defeat coronavirus, and make this information quickly publicly available to help other countries that would have to face a similar challenge.

DEVELOPMENT OF A CRITICAL CARE RESPONSE – CORONAVIRUS DISEASE 2019 LOMBARDY INTENSIVE CARE UNIT NETWORK ORGANIZATIONAL PERSPECTIVE

The critical care response to the COVID-19 pandemic started with the formation of an emergency task force on Feb. 21, created by the Lombardy region authorities and health care representatives: the COVID-19 Lombardy ICU Network (2). The aim of the COVID-19 Lombardy ICU Network was to manage the allocation of resources for all COVID-19 patients requiring ICU treatment in the region. The intensive care team of the Policlinico Maggiore Hospital in Milan led the clinical task force, which was active 24 hours per day, 7 days per week to manage bed request calls.

The 2 primary goals of the network in the initial response phase were to increase surge ICU capacity and to implement measures for containment.

Increase of Surge Intensive Care Unit Capacity

The precrisis ICU capacity was

- Lombardy: approximately 738 ICU beds (7.4 beds/100,000 people, equal to 2.9% of the total number of hospital beds)
- Italy: approximately 4682 ICU beds[4]

An exponential model for the prediction of ICU admission rate estimated a need of up to 2500 ICU beds in only 1 week for COVID-19 patients.[5] Using this model, the whole Italian National Health System would be saturated by mid-April. Drawing from the experience of the Venous-Venous ECMO Respiratory Failure Network,[6] one of the first initiatives of the network was to create 15 COVID-19 dedicated hub hospitals, with specific expertise in the management of patients with acute respiratory distress syndrome (ARDS) and infectious diseases.

Specific tasks of the hub hospitals were to:

1. Create dedicated ICU cohorts for COVID-19 patients
2. Create triage areas with the possibility to assist critical patients waiting for diagnostic test results for COVID-19

3. Establish local protocols for triage and rapid allocation of patients with respiratory symptoms
4. Ensure adequate personal protective equipment (PPE) availability and training of health care workers
5. Immediately notify the regional coordinating center of every confirmed case of critical COVID-19

Through a central coordination of the ICU Network, 130 ICU beds dedicated to COVID-19 patients were created in Lombardy in 48 hours. After the saturation of the designated hub hospitals, almost all hospitals of the region created dedicated ICUs, and on April 2, the ICU capacity reached 1750 beds. In addition, on March 31, 2020, the Milan Fair COVID-19 Intensive Care Hospital was inaugurated. The project, developed by Fondazione Fiera Milano in partnership with Lombardy Region consisted of a temporary hospital with up to 250 ICU beds developed in 20 days, and covering more than 25,000 square meters (**Fig. 1**). The hospital reorganization process, with the opening of newly dedicated ICUs, has been a multidisciplinary effort, with the involvement of health care providers, hospital managers, and political authorities.[7–9] The Italian government allocated 845 million euros to the National Health System to ensure a progressive increase of the number of ICU beds for invasive mechanical ventilation, up to 14% of the total hospital beds.[10]

Implementation of Measures for Containment

The government instituted extraordinary measures for containment: restrictions within lockdown areas (red zones) were implemented gradually, and then expanded to the entire country on March 9, 2020, until May 18, 2020. A second wave of infections is currently ongoing in several European countries, including Italy. Measures for containment and restrictions within Italian territory were instituted again from Oct. 26, 2020,

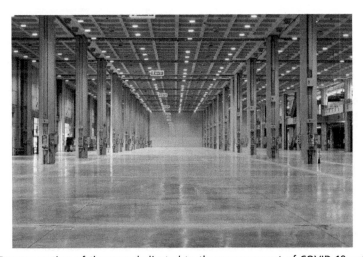

Fig. 1. Representation of the area dedicated to the management of COVID-19 patients at the Fair Milan Covid-19 Intensive Care Hospital covering more than 25,000 square meters of area Portello Pavilions 1 and 2 at Fieramilanocity, Milan, Italy. The image represents the empty space before Fair Milan Covid-19 Intensive Care Hospital was yet staged (permission obtained to reproduce the image by Fondazione Fiera – All Rights reserved – https://www.ospedalefieramilano.it/it/l-progetto.html).

based on the estimate of transmissibility within each region.[11] As of Dec. 13, 2020, the number of hospitalized patients in Lombardy and Italy was 5873 and 30,893, respectively; the number of ICU patients was 714 and 3,158, respectively. Overall, during the last 8 months, totals of 23,810 and 64,520 patients have died of SARS-CoV2 in Lombardy (**Fig. 2**A,B) and Italy (**Fig. 2**C,D), respectively.

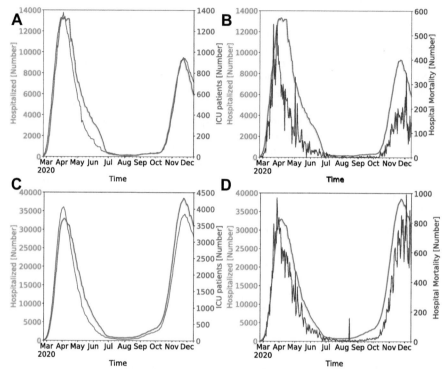

Fig. 2. Number of daily hospital versus ICU admissions (*A, C*) and hospital admissions versus hospital mortality (*B, D*) during the Italian first and second wave of SARS-CoV2 outbreak in Lombardy (top panels) and in Italy (bottom panels) from Feb. 24 to Dec. 13, 2020 (original data reports from the public source of "Presidenza del Consiglio dei Ministri - Dipartimento della Protezione Civile" https://github.com/pcm-dpc/COVID-19/blob/master/dati-regioni/dpc-covid19-ita-regioni.csv). (*D*) The peak of mortality reported on Aug. 15 was explained by internal verification of mortality data of Azienda Unità Sanitaria Locale of Parma (Emilia Romagna) that reported 154 deaths over March, April, and May that were not previously included. The distribution of hospitalized patients, ICU admissions, and deaths was different during the 2 peaks of the Italian SARS-CoV2 pandemic. In Lombardy, while the highest number of deaths during the first wave (ie, 546 deaths) was reported approximately 10 days before (ie, on March 20) the highest number of hospitalized patients (ie, 13,328 on April 4) and ICU admissions (ie, 1381 on April 3), during the second coronavirus peak, the highest capacitance in terms of hospital and ICU beds (ie, 9340 and 949, respectively) was reached earlier (ie, on Nov. 22), and contrary to the first wave, 10 days in advance compared with the highest number of deaths (ie, 347 on Dec. 3). Accordingly, in the whole country, a similar date was observed. During the first SARS-CoV2 wave, the highest number of deaths (ie, 969 deaths) was reported about 10 days before (ie, onMarch 26) compared with the highest request of hospital (ie, 33,004 on April 4) and ICU beds (ie, 4068 on April 3). In contrast, during the second peak of the pandemic, the highest numbers of hospital and ICU admissions (ie, 38,507 and 3848, respectively) were recorded on Nov. 23 and 25, respectively, about 10 days before the peak of COVID-19 deaths (ie, 993 on Dec. 3). (Visual courtesy of Francesco Casola.)

OUT-OF-HOSPITAL CORONAVIRUS DISEASE 2019 RESPONSE - AN ORGANIZATIONAL PERSPECTIVE
Organization of the Emergency Medical Service

The Emergency Medical Services (EMS) of the Lombardy region had to deal with an unprecedented increase in telephone calls to 112 (European emergency number) after the announcement of the first COVID-19 positive patient in Italy on Feb. 20, 2020. Call volumes registered a 264% increase compared with the 3 previous years on the 23rd of February in the metropolitan area of Milan (SOREU metropolitan).[12] Similar reports from other areas showed an increase in calls up to 440% compared with the pre-COVID-19 period.[13]

Several callers were just requesting information and guidance about COVID-19. Many others were suspected symptomatic patients deserving a prompt evaluation of respiratory symptoms, home isolation, and domicile SARS-CoV-2 testing or hospitalization. To cope with the escalation of calls, a COVID-19 response team was instituted by the EMS of the metropolitan area of Milan.[14] The team, composed of 10 health care professionals and 2 technicians, worked 24 hours per day 7 days per week in assessing the clinical condition of screened individuals to determine the need for hospital admission, or for home testing for SARS-CoV-2 and subsequent isolation. In essence, patients were screened for fever and any respiratory symptoms in order to

1. Organize ambulance
   dispatch and hospitalization in case of moderate or severe respiratory symptoms
2. Counsel, record, and isolate suspected or confirmed COVID-19 cases with mild symptoms

Despite efforts to maintain ordinary EMS activities through the creation of the COVID-19 response team, the reorganization of the 112 emergency response system, and the implementation of the staff, recent data showed that EMS arrival times were significantly higher compared with the same period in 2019 in Milan,[11] and in other provinces of Lombardy and Veneto, particularly for time-dependent conditions like out-of-hospital cardiac arrest.[15,16]

The Lombardy EMS coped with a dramatic increase in events caused by the outbreak in the region in an extremely short timeframe, and in a limited area, as occurred in the province of Bergamo. Data about the events managed by the dispatch center for the EMS of Brescia and Bergamo describe a devastating scenario. Fagoni and colleagues reported an increase of 50% in the number of events managed in March to April 2020, compared with the same period in 2019, with a tenfold increase in the number of the so-called respiratory or infective events. An alarming increase in the number of deaths was reported: +246% (odds ratio [OR] 1.7, $P<.0001$) in March to April 2020, compared with 2019.[17] This high mortality was in line with other reports from Italian cities severely affected by the COVID-19 pandemic in northern Italy.[18]

The Challenging Experience of Out-of-Hospital Cardiac Arrest During the Coronavirus Disease 2019 Outbreak

An almost 60% increase in out-of-hospital cardiac arrest (OHCA) incidence, coupled with a reduction in the short-term outcomes during the COVID-19 outbreak, was observed in Italy for the first time.[15] Specifically, during the first 40 days of the COVID-19 pandemic (Feb. 21 through March 31, 2020), the number of OHCAs occurring in the provinces of Lodi, Cremona, Pavia, and Mantua, increased up to 58% compared with the same period in 2019. An increase in the number of OHCA was seen in all 4 provinces, with a worrisome peak in the 2 most afflicted by COVID-19 infection: Lodi (+187%) and Cremona (+143%).

Among different etiologies, medical causes were more represented in OHCA during the COVID-19 pandemic. Age and sex of the patients were similar in the 2 study periods, but in 2020 home location and unwitnessed OHCA were more frequent compared with 2019. A decrease in bystander cardiopulmonary resuscitation rate of 15.6% was observed compared with the 2019 period. The median arrival time of emergency medical service was 3 minutes longer in 2020 than in 2019, and the incidence of out-of-hospital death was almost 15% higher in 2020 than in 2019. The cumulative incidence of out-of-hospital cardiac arrest in 2020 was strongly associated with the cumulative incidence of COVID-19. The authors then expanded the analysis to the following 60 days after the first COVID-19 patient was isolated, replicating the same results reported for the first 40 days.[19] On the contrary, a report from Padua in Veneto (northeast of Italy), did not highlight an increase in OHCA incidence and mortality.[16] However, in line with previous findings, the authors reported an increased EMS arrival time of 1.2 min in 2020 compared with 2019. Interestingly, when they broke the total arrival time into its main components (ie, call to dispatch, dispatch to departure, and departure to arrival), an increase in the time between the call and EMS departure was observed. The authors suggest that the longer call-to-departure time of the EMS could be due to the time spent to investigate COVID-19 status, while the delay in ambulance departure could be explained by PPE procedures and requirements.

IN-HOSPITAL CORONAVIRUS DISEASE 2019 RESPONSE - BUILDING SCIENTIFIC EVIDENCE
Intensive Care Unit Management of Coronavirus Disease 2019 Respiratory Failure

The COVID-19 Lombardy ICU Network was created to promptly respond to the SARS-CoV2 outbreak in Italy, and to manage the exponential surge of patients with respiratory failure, needing respiratory support in ICU. Fondazione IRCCS Ca' Granda Ospedale Maggiore Policlinico in Milan was the coordinating center of COVID-19 Lombardy ICU Network, which connected all the ICUs in the Lombardy region. Dedicated staff in the coordinator center of this consortium performed at least 2 telephone calls every day to obtain real-time granular information on most clinical characteristics and outcomes of patients admitted to the ICU.[20–22]

Despite the massive clinical and logistical efforts, COVID-19 Lombardy ICU Network was able to collect and provide scientific evidence about clinical characteristics, risk factors, pathophysiology, and prognosis of patients with SARS-CoV2 induced lung injury. Data collection was not limited to the mentioned phone calls, but also by local granular data collection in a centralized eCRF.

One of the aims of the COVID-19 Lombardy ICU Network was to deliver knowledge as rapidly as possible on a disease still poorly described, ultimately to help other countries facing a similarly dramatic health care experience.[23] Essentially, the research commitment of Ospedale Maggiore Policlinico was twofold in its objectives:

1. To build a registry that included all epidemiologic, clinical, and prognostic information of adult patients admitted to the hospital from the onset of the pandemic.
2. To create a biobank of samples to perform translational studies.

Data from this registry for national and international researchers will benefit patient care worldwide.[24] The authors summarized in **Table 1** the main scientific evidence reported by the COVID-19 Lombardy ICU Network, together with other Italian investigators, during the pandemic outbreak.

Table 1
Scientific evidence provided by the COVID-19 Lombardy ICU Network together with other Italian investigators during the pandemic outbreak to characterize the clinical history of critically ill COVID-19 patients

Areas of Research	Group of Research	Patient Population	Time of Inclusion	Main Findings
Clinical characteristics of COVID-19 ICU patients	COVID-19 Lombardy ICU Network[20]	1591 critically ill COVID-19 patients	Feb. 20 to March 8, 2020	• Median age of 63 (IQR 56–70) • Male-to-female ratio 4:1 • Hypertension was the most common comorbidity (49% of cases) • Of 1300 patients with ventilator data, 88% on mechanical ventilation, 11% on noninvasive ventilation • Median PEEP = 14 cmH$_2$O (IQR 12–16) -median Pao$_2$/Fio$_2$ = 160 (114–220) • Median Fio$_2$ = 70 (IQR 50–80) • Prone positioning was used in 27% of 875 patients • Patients with hypertension – compared to patients without hypertension – were older, with a more severe ARDS, requiring higher levels of PEEP and showing a higher ICU mortality (38 vs 22%, overall mortality 26%) • Short-term follow-up and half of patients with complete data at follow-up (March 25, 2020) were still in ICU

(continued on next page)

Table 1
(continued)

Areas of Research	Group of Research	Patient Population	Time of Inclusion	Main Findings
Risk factors of mortality in COVID-19 ICU patients	COVID-19 Lombardy ICU Network[21]	3988 critically ill COVID-19 patients	Feb. 20 to April 22	• Mortality was higher in males; in patients with at least 1 comorbidity; and in older patients (56 years old was the cut off – follow-up until May 30) • A higher severity of lung injury (ie, patients with a lower Pao_2, a higher Fio_2, and higher PEEP levels [$\geq$13 cmH$_2$O]) and a shorter duration of mechanical ventilation and hospital length of stay were correlated with a higher mortality rate • Among independent predictors of mortality – adjusted for time effect – 1. Older age and male sex (ie, baseline characteristics); 2. Hypercholesterolemia, type 2 diabetes, and chronic obstructive pulmonary disease (COPD) (ie, comorbidities); 3. A higher PEEP, a higher Fio_2 and a lower Pao_2/Fio_2 at admission (severity of lung injury); and 4. A trend to the use of any mechanical respiratory support (either noninvasive or invasive) was associated with a higher mortality rate

| Pathophysiology of COVID-19 ARDS patients | Grasselli et al,[22] 2020 | 301 critically ill COVID-19 patients | March 9 -22 | 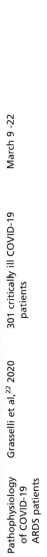<ul><li>Prospective multicenter observational study conducted in different regions from north to south of Italy</li><li>Median respiratory system compliance was 9 mL/cmH$_2$O higher in COVID-19 associated ARDS compared to patients with ARDS unrelated to COVID-19</li><li>Lung injury associated to COVID-19 appeared not only to be characterized by a parenchymal damage but included also an endothelial injury</li><li>The study reported a strong association between D-dimer concentration and areas of pulmonary hypoperfusion that was assessed by computed tomography (CT)-pulmonary angiography in a subgroup of patients</li><li>The role of different combination of levels of respiratory system compliance and D-dimer on outcome was investigated - in a multivariate model adjusted for sex, age, and severity of ARDS using Pao$_2$/Fio$_2$ the group of patients at the higher risk of mortality was the one with the worse epithelial and endothelial lung injury, as suggested by the combination of high D-dimer concentration and low compliance of the respiratory system</li></ul> |

(continued on next page)

Table 1
(continued)

Areas of Research	Group of Research	Patient Population	Time of Inclusion	Main Findings
Hematological characteristics of COVID-19 patients	• Angelo Bianchi Bonomi Hemophilia and Thrombosis Center in Milan (COHERENT project)[25] • Angelo Bianchi Bonomi Hemophilia and Thrombosis Center in Milan[26]	• 62 COVID-19 patients – with low, intermediate or high intensity of care • 24 critically ill COVID-19 patients	First peak of the Italian COVID-19 outbreak	Both studies – according to the analyses of laboratory biomarkers of pro and anticoagulation, together with data regarding the viscoelastic properties of blood of COVID-19 patients by the use of thromboelastography – do not support hematological characteristics of disseminated intravascular coagulation – in contrast they demonstrated the presence of a prothrombotic phenotype that leads to a procoagulant imbalance that originates from a complex interplay between the inflammatory insult, hemostasis, and endothelial cells perturbation

Double patient ventilation with a single ventilator – feasible and ethical?

During a pandemic, there may be an imbalance between the numbers of critically ill patients requiring invasive ventilation, and the numbers of mechanical ventilators that are available. An interesting option that was proposed almost 15 years ago by Neyman and Irvin is to connect multiple patients to a single ventilator in order to compensate for the equipment shortage.[27] Researchers from Milano and Bologna in Italy successfully tested the feasibility of using a single turbine ventilator to provide ventilation in 2 simulated patients with different respiratory mechanic characteristics.[28] Beitler and colleagues took this experience to the next level and provided evidence of feasibility in COVID-19 patients with ARDS who shared ventilators for at least 2 days, under rigorous protocols, and experienced no adverse events.[29] This strategy still remains experimental. Critical points still need to be addressed such as the matching of respiratory mechanic characteristics of patients ventilated with a single ventilator – in order to avoid harm in one of them - and the safety of prolonged ventilator sharing.

Out of Intensive Care Unit Management of Coronavirus Disease 2019 Respiratory Failure

Noninvasive ventilation – state-of-the-art and guidelines

As stated, the massive burden of SARS-CoV2 on the Italian health care system quickly saturated the availability of ICU beds and mechanical ventilators. Among several, one of the challenges for health care providers was to manage and contain severe intrahospital respiratory failure outside the critical care environment. Noninvasive ventilation allowed physicians to stabilize patients, avoiding the progression to severe hypoxemia and muscle exhaustion that would eventually require invasive mechanical ventilation. Noninvasive positive pressure oxygenation strategies have been recently confirmed to be associated with a lower mortality risk compared to standard oxygen therapy.[30]

Noninvasive positive pressure ventilation (NIPPV) has played a key role in the management of COVID-19 patients out of the ICU during the Italian crisis surge. The rapid guidelines of the European Society of Intensive Care Medicine suggested on 1 side high-flow nasal cannula (HFNC) and NIPPV as strategies to reduce the need for intubation and overcome shortages of mechanical ventilators; on the other side, NIPPV was suggested for invasive ventilation as a last option in a scenario of a shortage of standard full-featured ventilators.[31] The worldwide guidelines on the management of critically ill COVID-19 patients confirmed the suggestion of the implementation of HFNC and NIPPV in acute hypoxemic respiratory failure (AHRF) and recommended early intubation in a controlled setting if worsening occurred.[32] The potential increase of virus aerosolization with NIPPV remains a significant concern regarding transmission of infection to health care providers.[33]

The Italian helmet continuous positive airway pressure experience during the coronavirus disease pandemic

The Italian approach to noninvasive ventilator management of COVID-19 AHRF was characterized in northern Italy by the use of helmet continuous positive airway pressure (c-PAP), because of the large Italian experience in the management of AHRF with this interface.[34]

The helmet is an interface of utmost utility in a pandemic scenario, in order to avoid the risk of aerosolization when helmet NIPPV is delivered through a ventilator, as suggested by Cabrini and colleagues[35] However, the use of helmet c-PAP has an excellent performance simply with a free-flow generator and a positive end-expiratory pressure (PEEP) valve at the helmet outlet, combined with a high-efficiency particulate air (HEPA) filter at the helmet outlet to reduce the risk of environmental contamination.[31,36] Furthermore, the helmet c-PAP bundle was proposed to optimize patient comfort using

1. A heat and moisture exchanger (HME) filter to decrease incoming noise
2. Counterweight fixing systems to stabilize the helmet position
3. Heated wire tubing with active humidification[37]

Early consensus management of non-ICU patients with SARS-CoV2 in Italy suggested the use of helmet c-PAP without humidification as the first choice.[38] Three Italian studies have reported data on the use of helmet c-PAP and NIPPV out of a critical care environment in COVID-19 patients.[39–41]

1. In a multicenter observational prospective study, Aliberti and colleagues described the characteristics and the outcome of patients undergoing c-PAP treatment in 3 high-dependency units in 2 Italian hospitals in Milan during the first pandemic wave. Out of 157 patients, helmet c-PAP successfully improved oxygenation from a Pao_2/Fio_2 = 143 to 206. However, intubation or death was higher compared to non-COVID-19 patients with the same severity of AHRF (45% vs 23%). Interestingly, patients with c-PAP failure showed higher inflammation (eg, high interleukin [IL]-6 levels) and activation of the coagulation cascade (eg, high D-Dimer levels) compared with patients who did not fail helmet c-PAP.[39]

2. In the emergency department of Papa Giovanni XXIII hospital (HPG23) from Bergamo (a city overly affected by the surge), Duca and colleagues described patient characteristics and the ventilator management. In a time frame of 10 days, the authors reported that out of 611 patients admitted to the emergency department with suspected COVID-19, 99 received ventilator support (12% invasive and 88% noninvasive) in the emergency department, and 85 of them were confirmed positive to SARS-CoV2 (median age 70 years, median Pao_2/Fio_2 ratio = 128). Given the resource limitation in the ICU setting at the outbreak onset, the internal hospital protocol in the emergency department of HPG23 adopted the use of helmet c-PAP or NIPPV in the presence of hypoxemia (SpO2<90%) or RR greater than 30/min during the administration of oxygen therapy by non-rebreather mask with an oxygen flow of 15 L/min. Patients were admitted to the ward until availability of an ICU bed. The follow-up mortality 2 months later was 77%, which was potentially explained by the severity of hypoxemia of patients admitted to the emergency department with standard oxygen therapy already maximized.[40]

3. The results from the largest data set that described the prevalence and the clinical characteristics of patients with COVID-19 treated with NIV outside the ICU, and that explored the factors associated with NIV failure (defined as need of intubation or death) were reported by Bellani and colleagues in a prospective single-day prevalence study (WARd-COVID). In 31 centers within the COVID-19 Lombardy ICU Network 8753 COVID-19 patients were present, accounting for an average of 62% of the overall hospital beds. Of these, 909 subjects (10.4%) received NIV out of the ICU. The use of the helmet or face-mask was used in a ratio of 3:1. NIV failed in 300 patients (37.6%). A higher c-reactive protein and lower Pao_2/Fio_2 and platelet counts were independent predictors of NIV failure. Mortality rate was 25% at 60-day follow-up. Although with a large sample size and the multicentric design of the study, the lower rates of NIV failure and mortality in the WARd-COVID – compared with previous reported studies[39,40] - may be explained by the different timing of patient enrollment and data collection (ie, 1 month later that the Italian SARS-CoV2 outbreak). At that time, the organizational optimization

of the ICU resources was already implemented by the COVID-19 Lombardy ICU Network. This consisted of an exponential increase of the number of ICU beds that might have allowed to treat patients with a less severe acute hypercapnic respiratory failure (AHRF) on the ward at the moment of patient enrollment (average $Pa_{O_2}/Fi_{O_2} = 168$).[41] An exemplary image representing the use of helmet c-PAP in prone positioning – as performed in the authors' Institutions in Monza and Milano – is provided in **Fig. 3**.

The Italian experience with prone-positioning in spontaneously breathing patients
As with ARDS from other causes,[42] COVID-19 guidelines propose cycles of 12 to 16 hours of prone positioning in patients with moderate-severe ARDS and undergoing mechanical ventilation,[33] based on strong physiologic rationale.[43,44] No information was provided on the use of proning in awake, non-intubated patients in the recent guidelines where the knowledge of the benefits is limited. Nonsystematic differences have been reported in prone positioning compared to supine positioning in healthy volunteers, with the presence of a more homogeneous perfusion in selected subjects that might improve ventilation/perfusion matching.[45] The use of PEEP has been described to increase the ventilation/perfusion ratio in the dorsal areas of healthy subjects.[46] However, little is known in terms of the physiologic effects of PEEP in patients undergoing prone positioning with a severe impairment of gas exchange, as in the case with COVID-19 related ARDS.

Italy pioneered the use of prone positioning in awake COVID-19 patients spontaneously breathing and explored the role of noninvasive ventilation during protonation outside the ICU.

1. In a prospective study, Coppo and colleagues explored the feasibility and physiologic effects of prone positioning in 56 patients - on supplemental oxygen therapy only (21%) or with helmet c-PAP (79%). Prone positioning was feasible in 84% of patients. Oxygenation was significantly improved in the prone position (average Pa_{O_2}/Fi_{O_2}, 286 vs 181, $P<.0001$), and the oxygenation gain was maintained in 50% of the patient population after resupination. Among other factors, prone positioning seemed more effective if applied early after hospital admission.[47]
2. Data from a retrospective study by Ramirez and colleagues reported that pronation was feasible outside the ICU. Furthermore, patient mobilization, which included prone positioning, was effective in reducing failure rates of c-PAP in COVID-19 patients.[48]

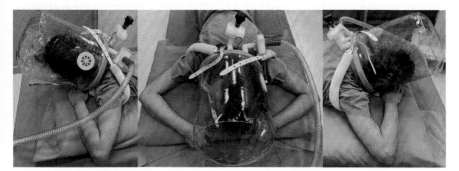

Fig. 3. Exemplary image of continuous positive pressure ventilation delivered by a helmet c-PAP during prone positioning in a healthy volunteer as per the authors' practice at San Gerardo Hospital, Monza and Policlinico Maggiore Hospital, Milano.

3. Bastoni and colleagues reported a series of 10 patients who met criteria for proning. In 6 patients, with a median Pao_2/Fio_2 of 68 mm Hg, prone positioning was effective at increasing oxygenation to a median Pao_2/Fio_2 of 97 mm Hg 1 hour after.[49]
4. The use of both prone and lateral positioning for 1 hour has been tested in 26 COVID-19 patients during helmet c-PAP admitted to the high-dependency unit of Policlinico Hospital in Milan. Retucci and colleagues observed that the success rate (ie, oxygenation improvement) of proning was higher compared with the use of lateral positioning. However, the short duration of patient positioning may have contributed to the loss of the beneficial improvement of oxygenation when patients returned to the semiseated position.[50]

In-hospital interplay and differences in the use of critical care resources between critical and noncritical care environments

Three regions in northern Italy joined together in a common effort to build a large network that included different experiences from the part of Italy that was severely hit by the outbreak. This led to the development of the COVID-19 Northern Italian ICU Network, which strived to report scientific evidence on the management and patient characteristics from different Italian areas.

In an interesting analysis from the COVID-19 Northern Italian ICU Network, the investigators reported differences among patients managed in and out of the ICU during the first 14 days of the pandemic outbreak (Feb. 24 to March 8, 2020). In the ICU, bed capacity rapidly increased from 1545 to 1989 beds (28.7%). In data obtained in 802 patients within 14 days, the percentage of patients who received respiratory support increased from 0.6% to 37% out of the ICU. Patients were located in the infectious disease ward, pneumology ward, emergency medicine, and intermediate care unit, with a proportion of 47%, 31%, 15%, and 7%, respectively. The proportion of patients admitted to ICU decreased from 20.3% to 15.2%. Patients located out of the ICU, compared to within the ICU, had more comorbidities, received more oxygen therapy and NIV, (with the exception of c-PAP that did not differ between the 2 groups), had higher Pao_2/Fio_2 and pH, and lower respiratory rate, $Paco_2$, and base excess.[3]

A useful score to predict clinical deterioration (defined as escalation of care to the ICU or death) in COVID-19 patients was proposed by Cecconi and colleagues. Higher levels of C-reactive protein (CRP) and creatinine, together with the presence of coronary artery disease, higher degree of hypoxemia, and a respiratory rate above or equal to 20 breaths per minute were used to build a prognostic index with a high predictive accuracy (85%) and easy implementation at bedside.[51] The findings obtained by Cecconi and coworkers were confirmed by the CORIST study – including almost 4000 patients from 30 clinical centers from northern, central and southern Italy – in which elevated CRP, impaired renal function, and advanced age predicted in-hospital mortality.[52]

SURGICAL PROCEDURES – CORONAVIRUS DISEASE 2019 POSITIVE AND NEGATIVE PATIENTS

The hospital overload of COVID-19 patients led to a sudden and unplanned interruption of elective surgical activities that led to the difficult process of balancing between the risk of delaying a cancer diagnosis and treatment, versus suffering a potential COVID-19 exposure, An individualized approach, based on a case-by case evaluation, is suggested.[53] Furthermore, in COVID-19-positive patients, precise, well-established plans and protocols must be implemented to perform emergent and nondeferrable surgical procedures.[54]

NATIONAL GUIDELINES ON RESOURCE ALLOCATION DURING CORONAVIRUS DISEASE 2019 – THE RESPONSE OF THE ITALIAN SOCIETY OF ANESTHESIA, ANALGESIA, RESUSCITATION, AND INTENSIVE CARE

The Italian Society of Anesthesia, Analgesia, Resuscitation, and Intensive Care (SIAARTI) provided documents and recommendations to manage the SARS-CoV2 outbreak at different levels, including both clinical practice[55] and ethical considerations.[56,57]

From an ethical perspective, SIAARTI elaborated recommendations in a scenario in which the surge of critical patients admitted to the hospital created an "imbalance between the real clinical needs of the population and the effective availability of intensive resources." The society highlighted 3 principles that should guide the decision-making process for appropriate allocation of limited health care resources:

1. Clinical appropriateness
2. Proportionality of care
3. Distributive justice

The SIAARTI guidelines aimed to help the clinicians in managing the potential emotional burden associated with resource allocation and make explicit the criteria for resource allocation. Although individual judgment must be considered part of the clinical decision, the presence of national recommendations served as a guide for clinicians to avoid frank disparities in the judgment and an arbitrary perspective in the presence of dramatic choices.

Scarce resources should be evaluated and considered in the presence of a higher probability of survival and of saved years of life – evaluating patient age, comorbidities, and the functional status before the event – and aiming to achieve a better outcome for the highest number of people.[56,57] Ethical and legal nuances of the national recommendations have been provided by the SIAARTI.[58,59]

SIAARTI, with the collaboration of Società Italiana di Infermieri di Terapia Intensiva (ANIARTI), Società Italiana di Medicina di Emergenza e Urgenza (SIMEU), Società Italiana di Cure Palliative (SICP), also provided guidance to health care workers for the management of communication on patient clinical conditions to the families that were completely isolated during the lockdown, and could not have any visual or physical interaction with their relative admitted to the hospital. The document, shared by these 4 societies, had 3 components, including a statement on communication with families, the key points used to develop the statements, and a checklist with instructions for how to make appropriate phone calls.[60]

Communication of clinical information to patient families was made difficult not only by the severity and acuity of such a novel disease, but also by the fear of the disease in non-health care workers, which created situations where health care professionals were praised while they were at work, but experienced discrimination when outside of the hospital setting.[61] This may have contributed to a psychological effect in the frontline personnel of the SARS-CoV2 pandemic.[62]

To promote awareness among people about the clinical condition of patients, and the daily working conditions of the health care workers during the COVID outbreak in Italy, Hope Onlus was created in collaboration with the Ospedale Maggiore Policlinico in Milan, and promoted the project "#Covid-19 con Hope" #Covid-19@storiedisperanza (www.hopeonlus.org). This important project has an educational and cultural mandate to explain the impact of COVID-19 on the society to Italian citizens within a humanitarian program of Hope Onlus, at both national and international levels. This project is composed of photo exhibitions, including images of the real-life conditions in the hospitals, together with stories of the health care workers in action (**Fig. 4**). The

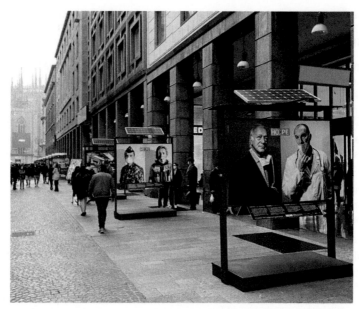

Fig. 4. Humanitarian Program Hope Onlus "#Covid-19 con Hope" #Covid-19@storiedisper-anza. On the first stand, Prof. Antonio Pesenti, on the left, and Prof. Giacomo Grasselli, on the right – Clinical Director and Clinical Lead of the Intensive Care Unit of Policlinico Maggiore Hospital, Milano – the 2 main actors who led the Lombardy Crisis Unit and coordinated the COVID-19 Lombardy ICU network.

authors' university is also participating in the FLOWS project, led by the National University of Ireland in Galway, which aims to identify the needs and development of best practice guidance for the psychological support of frontline health care workers during and after COVID-19.[63]

In conclusion, the Italian critical care experience during the first wave of the COVID-19 pandemic was a pioneer example of an organizational and clinical response to the outbreak. At the same time, a continuous effort was made to provide scientific evidence to understand how to better defeat coronavirus, and make this information available to help other countries worldwide.

CLINICS CARE POINTS

- Italy was the first western country to face a large COVID-19 outbreak.
- COVID19 Lombardy Network responded to the surge of hospital admissions in the Northern Italy; it organized a rapid increase in ICU beds and implemented measures for containment.
- Scientific evidence was provided by Italian centers to characterize the clinical history of COVID-19 associated respiratory failure
- Relevant experience was collected in Italy during the pandemic about the use of noninvasive continuous positive airway pressure and awake proning, which were remarkably implemented to manage respiratory failure out of the ICU setting.
- Recommendations from national guidelines were structured to guide health care providers on resource allocation; promotion of awareness among Italian citizens within specific humanitarian and educational programs was implemented

ACKNOWLEDGMENTS

The authors thank Francesco Casola, PhD, for his help with the visual of **Fig. 2**.

DISCLOSURE

The authors have nothing to disclose.

REFERENCES

1. WHO Director-General's opening remarks at the media briefing on COVID-19: 11 March 2020. 2020. Available at: https://covid19.who.int/?gclid=Cj0KCQiA-OeBBhDiARIsADyBcE4_O7cTc98_eNV7hXefnM_DNAfVfCmwKaXlmvzHipvRpqTFmrlaGBsaAq0VEALw_wcB.
2. Grasselli G, Pesenti A, Cecconi M. Critical care utilization for the COVID-19 outbreak in Lombardy, Italy: early experience and forecast during an emergency response. JAMA 2020;323(16):1545–6.
3. Tonetti T, Grasselli G, Zanella A, et al. Use of critical care resources during the first 2 weeks (February 24-March 8, 2020) of the Covid-19 outbreak in Italy. Ann Intensive Care 2020;10(1):133.
4. Pecoraro F, Clemente F, Luzi D. The efficiency in the ordinary hospital bed management in Italy: An in-depth analysis of intensive care unit in the areas affected by COVID-19 before the outbreak. PLoS One 2020;15(9):e0239249.
5. Remuzzi A, Remuzzi G. COVID-19 and Italy: what next? Lancet 2020;395(10231): 1225–8.
6. Patroniti N, Zangrillo A, Pappalardo F, et al. The Italian ECMO network experience during the 2009 influenza A(H1N1) pandemic: preparation for severe respiratory emergency outbreaks. Intensive Care Med 2011;37(9):1447–57.
7. Fagiuoli S, Lorini FL, Remuzzi G, et al. Adaptations and Lessons in the Province of Bergamo. N Engl J Med 2020;382(21):e71.
8. Carenzo L, Costantini E, Greco M, et al. Hospital surge capacity in a tertiary emergency referral centre during the COVID-19 outbreak in Italy. Anaesthesia 2020;75(7):928–34.
9. Buoro S, Di Marco F, Rizzi M, et al. Papa Giovanni XXIII Bergamo Hospital at the time of the COVID-19 outbreak: Letter from the warfront. Int J Lab Hematol 2020; 42(Suppl 1):8–10.
10. Available at: https://www.gazzettaufficiale.it/eli/id/2020/03/09/20G00030/sg. Accessed December 13, 2020.
11. Cori A, Ferguson NM, Fraser C, et al. A new framework and software to estimate time-varying reproduction numbers during epidemics. Am J Epidemiol 2013; 178(9):1505–12.
12. Marrazzo F, Spina S, Pepe PE, et al. Rapid reorganization of the Milan metropolitan public safety answering point operations during the initial phase of the COVID-19 outbreak in Italy. J Am Coll Emerg Physicians Open 2020;1(6):1240–9.
13. Perlini S, Canevari F, Cortesi S, et al. Emergency department and out-of-hospital emergency system (112-AREU 118) integrated response to coronavirus disease 2019 in a northern Italy centre. Intern Emerg Med 2020;15(5):825–33.
14. Spina S, Marrazzo F, Migliari M, et al. The response of Milan's emergency medical system to the COVID-19 outbreak in Italy. Lancet 2020;395(10227):e49–50.
15. Baldi E, Sechi GM, Mare C, et al. Out-of-hospital cardiac arrest during the covid-19 outbreak in Italy. N Engl J Med 2020;383(5):496–8.

16. Paoli A, Brischigliaro L, Squizzato T, et al. Out-of-hospital cardiac arrest during the COVID-19 pandemic in the Province of Padua, Northeast Italy. Resuscitation 2020;154:47–9.

17. Fagoni N, Perone G, Villa GF, et al. The Lombardy emergency medical system faced with COVID-19: the impact of out-of-hospital outbreak. Prehosp Emerg Care 2020;25:1–7.

18. Piccininni M, Rohmann JL, Foresti L, et al. Use of all cause mortality to quantify the consequences of covid-19 in Nembro, Lombardy: descriptive study. BMJ 2020;369:m1835.

19. Baldi E, Sechi GM, Mare C, et al. COVID-19 kills at home: the close relationship between the epidemic and the increase of out-of-hospital cardiac arrests. Eur Heart J 2020;41(32):3045–54.

20. Grasselli G, Zangrillo A, Zanella A, et al. Baseline characteristics and outcomes of 1591 patients infected with SARS-CoV-2 Admitted to ICUs of the lombardy region, Italy. JAMA 2020;323(16):1574–81.

21. Grasselli G, Greco M, Zanella A, et al. Risk factors associated with mortality among patients with COVID-19 in intensive care units in Lombardy, Italy. JAMA Intern Med 2020;180(10):1–11.

22. Grasselli G, Tonetti T, Protti A, et al. Pathophysiology of COVID-19-associated acute respiratory distress syndrome: a multicentre prospective observational study. Lancet Respir Med 2020;8(12):1201–8.

23. Cook DJ, Marshall JC, Fowler RA. Critical illness in patients with COVID-19: mounting an effective clinical and research response. JAMA 2020;323(16): 1559–60.

24. Bandera A, Aliberti S, Gualtierotti R, et al. Response of an Italian reference institute to research challenges regarding a new pandemic: COVID-19 network. Clin Microbiol Infect 2020;S1198-743X(20):30374–8.

25. Peyvandi F, Artoni A, Novembrino C, et al. Hemostatic alterations in COVID-19. Haematologica 2020. https://doi.org/10.3324/haematol.2020.262634.

26. Panigada M, Bottino N, Tagliabue P, et al. Hypercoagulability of COVID-19 patients in intensive care unit: a report of thromboelastography findings and other parameters of hemostasis. J Thromb Haemost 2020;18(7):1738–42.

27. Neyman G, Irvin CB. A single ventilator for multiple simulated patients to meet disaster surge. Acad Emerg Med 2006;13:1246–9.

28. Tonetti T, Zanella A, Pizzilli G, et al. One ventilator for two patients: feasibility and considerations of a last resort solution in case of equipment shortage. Thorax 2020;75(6):517–9.

29. Beitler JR, Mittel AM, Kallet R, et al. Ventilator sharing during an acute shortage caused by the COVID-19 pandemic. Am J Respir Crit Care Med 2020;202(4): 600–4.

30. Ferreyro BL, Angriman F, Munshi L, et al. Association of noninvasive oxygenation strategies with all-cause mortality in adults with acute hypoxemic respiratory failure: a systematic review and meta-analysis. JAMA 2020;324(1):57–67.

31. Aziz S, Arabi YM, Alhazzani W, et al. Managing ICU surge during the COVID-19 crisis: rapid guidelines. Intensive Care Med 2020;46(7):1303–25.

32. Alhazzani W, Møller MH, Arabi YM, et al. Surviving sepsis campaign: guidelines on the management of critically ill adults with coronavirus disease 2019 (COVID-19). Intensive Care Med 2020;46(5):854–87.

33. Hui DS, Chow BK, Ng SS, et al. Exhaled air dispersion distances during noninvasive ventilation via different Respironics face masks. Chest 2009;136:998–1005.

34. Bellani G, Patroniti N, Greco M, et al. The use of helmets to deliver non-invasive continuous positive airway pressure in hypoxemic acute respiratory failure. Minerva Anestesiol 2008;74(11):651–6.

35. Cabrini L, Landoni G, Zangrillo A. Minimise nosocomial spread of 2019-nCoV when treating acute respiratory failure. Lancet 2020;395(10225):685.

36. Lucchini A, Giani M, Winterton D, et al. Procedures to minimize viral diffusion in the intensive care unit during the COVID-19 pandemic. Intensive Crit Care Nurs 2020;60:102894.

37. Lucchini A, Giani M, Isgrò S, et al. The "helmet bundle" in COVID-19 patients undergoing non invasive ventilation. Intensive Crit Care Nurs 2020;58:102859.

38. Vitacca M, Nava S, Santus P, et al. Early consensus management for non-ICU ARF SARS-CoV-2 emergency in Italy: from ward to trenches. Eur Respir J 2020;55(5):2000632.

39. Aliberti S, Radovanovic D, Billi F, et al. Helmet CPAP treatment in patients with COVID-19 pneumonia: a multicenter, cohort study. Eur Respir J 2020;56(4):2001935.

40. Duca A, Memaj I, Zanardi F, et al. Severity of respiratory failure and outcome of patients needing a ventilatory support in the Emergency Department during Italian novel coronavirus SARS-CoV2 outbreak: preliminary data on the role of Helmet CPAP and non-invasive positive pressure ventilation. EClinicalMedicine 2020;24:100419.

41. Bellani G, Grasselli G, Cecconi M, et al. Noninvasive ventilatory support of COVID-19 patients outside the Intensive Care Units (WARd-COVID). Ann Am Thorac Soc 2021. https://doi.org/10.1513/AnnalsATS.202008-1080OC.

42. Fan E, Del Sorbo L, Goligher EC, et al. An Official American Thoracic Society/European Society of Intensive Care Medicine/Society of Critical Care Medicine clinical practice guideline: mechanical ventilation in adult patients with acute respiratory distress syndrome. Am J Respir Crit Care Med 2017;195(9):1253–63.

43. Gattinoni L, Taccone P, Carlesso E, et al. Prone position in acute respiratory distress syndrome. Rationale, indications, and limits. Am J Respir Crit Care Med 2013;188(11):1286–93.

44. Guerin C, Baboi L, Richard JC. Mechanisms of the effects of prone positioning in acute respiratory distress syndrome. Intensive Care Med 2014;40(11):1634–42.

45. Musch G, Layfield JDH, Harris RS, et al. Topographical distribution of pulmonary perfusion and ventilation, assessed by PET in supine and prone humans. J Appl Physiol (1985) 2002;93(5):1841–51.

46. Mure M, Nyrén S, Jacobsson H, et al. High continuous positive airway pressure level induces ventilation/perfusion mismatch in the prone position. Crit Care Med 2001;29(5):959–64.

47. Coppo A, Bellani G, Winterton D, et al. Feasibility and physiological effects of prone positioning in non-intubated patients with acute respiratory failure due to COVID-19 (PRON-COVID): a prospective cohort study. Lancet Respir Med 2020;8(8):765–74.

48. Ramirez GA, Bozzolo EP, Castelli E, et al. Continuous positive airway pressure and pronation outside the intensive care unit in COVID 19 ARDS. Minerva Med 2020. https://doi.org/10.23736/S0026-4806.20.06952-9.

49. Bastoni D, Poggiali E, Vercelli A, et al. Prone positioning in patients treated with non-invasive ventilation for COVID-19 pneumonia in an Italian emergency department. Emerg Med J 2020;37(9):565–6.

50. Retucci M, Aliberti S, Ceruti C, et al. Prone and lateral positioning in spontaneously breathing patients with COVID-19 pneumonia undergoing noninvasive helmet CPAP Treatment. Chest 2020;158(6):2431–5.
51. Cecconi M, Piovani D, Brunetta E, et al. Early predictors of clinical deterioration in a cohort of 239 patients hospitalized for COVID-19 infection in Lombardy, Italy. J Clin Med 2020;9(5):1548.
52. Di Castelnuovo A, Bonaccio M, Costanzo S, et al. Common cardiovascular risk factors and in-hospital mortality in 3,894 patients with COVID-19: survival analysis and machine learning-based findings from the multicentre Italian CORIST Study. Nutr Metab Cardiovasc Dis 2020;30(11):1899–913.
53. Moletta L, Sefora Pierobon E, Capovilla G, et al. International guidelines and recommendations for surgery during COVID-19 pandemic: a systematic review. Int J Surg 2020;79:180–8.
54. Coccolini F, Perrone G, Chiarugi M, et al. Surgery in COVID-19 patients: operational directives. World J Emerg Surg 2020;15(1):25.
55. Sorbello M, El-Boghdadly K, Di Giacinto I, et al. The Italian coronavirus disease 2019 outbreak: recommendations from clinical practice. Anaesthesia 2020;75(6):724–32.
56. Vergano M, Bertolini G, Giannini A, et al. SIAARTI recommendations for the allocation of intensive care treatments in exceptional, resource-limited circumstances. Minerva Anestesiol 2020;86(5):469–72.
57. Vergano M, Bertolini G, Giannini A, et al. Clinical ethics recommendations for the allocation of intensive care treatments in exceptional, resource-limited circumstances: The Italian perspective during the COVID-19 epidemic. Crit Care 2020;24:165.
58. Piccinni M, Aprile A, Benciolini P, et al. [Ethical, deontologic and legal considerations about SIAARTI document "clinical ethics recommendations for the allocation of intensive care treatments, in exceptional, resource-limited circumstances." Recenti Prog Med 2020;111(4):212–22.
59. Sulmasy DP. Principled decisions and virtuous care: an ethical assessment of the SIAARTI Guidelines for allocating intensive care resources. Minerva Anestesiol 2020;86(8):872–6.
60. Multidisciplinary Working Group. ComuniCovid." Italian Society of Anesthesia and Intensive Care (SIAARTI), Italian Association of Critical Care Nurses (Aniarti), ItalianSociety of Emergency Medicine (SIMEU), and Italian SocietyPalliative Care (SICP). How to communicate with families of patients in complete isolation during SARS-CoV-2 pandemic multidisciplinary working group "ComuniCoViD. Recenti Prog Med 2020;111(6):357–67.
61. Cabrini L, Grasselli G, Cecconi M, et al. Yesterday heroes, today plague doctors: the dark side of celebration. Intensive Care Med 2020;46(9):1790–1.
62. Azoulay E, De Waele J, Ferrer R, et al. Symptoms of burnout in intensive care unit specialists facing the COVID-19 outbreak. Ann Intensive Care 2020;10(1):110.
63. Available at: https://hrbopenresearch.org/articles/3-54. Accessed December 13, 2020.

Anesthesiology and Critical Care Response to COVID-19 in Resource-Limited Settings

Experiences from Nepal

Gentle S. Shrestha, MD, EDIC, FCCP, FNCS[a,*], Ritesh Lamsal, MD, DM[a],
Pradip Tiwari, MD[b], Subhash P. Acharya, MD, FCCP[a]

KEYWORDS

- Anesthesiology • Critical care • COVID-19 • Nepal • Resource-limited

KEY POINTS

- Most of the world's population does not have access to safe and affordable surgical and anesthesia care.
- Anesthesia and critical care delivery systems in resource-limited settings grappling to manage patients have been overwhelmed by the current COVID-19 pandemic.
- Evidence derived from high-income countries and international guidelines on COVID-19 cannot be easily implemented or may not be applicable in resource-limited settings.
- Low- and middle-income countries must perform high-quality indigenous research, use innovative measures, determine minimal standards of care, and focus on attainable clinical goals.

INTRODUCTION

As the human population continues to rise, the global burden of surgical procedures and the need for anesthesia and critical care is increasing. According to the World Health Organization, the global burden of surgeries was more than 310 million in 2012, with an increase of nearly 40% from a similar estimate in 2004.[1] A recent report highlighted that nearly 5 billion people do not have access to safe, affordable surgical and anesthesia care, and one-third of the global burden of disease requires surgery and anesthesia management.[2] However, only a small number of surgeries are carried out in low- and middle-income countries (LMICs), mainly because of the lack of

[a] Department of Anaesthesiology, Tribhuvan University Teaching Hospital, Maharajgunj Road, PO Box: 1524, Maharajgunj, Kathmandu 44600, Nepal; [b] Department of Critical Care, Norvic International Hospital, PO Box: 14126, Thapathali, Kathmandu 44617, Nepal
* Corresponding author.
E-mail address: gentlesunder@hotmail.com

Anesthesiology Clin 39 (2021) 285–292
https://doi.org/10.1016/j.anclin.2021.02.004   **anesthesiology.theclinics.com**

resources and personnel. The disparity in the distribution of health care among countries will probably widen in the near future, because LMICs have a higher population growth compared with high-income countries.

The pandemic of COVID-19 is evolving. The spectrum of COVID-19 varies from asymptomatic cases to severe disease requiring intensive care admission and multiorgan support. Nearly 80% of COVID-19 patients experience mild-to-moderate symptoms and around 5% of cases require intensive care unit (ICU) admission.[3] However, the distribution and severity of COVID-19 are substantially dissimilar in different parts of the world. The mortality rate of cases admitted to the ICU is between 23.4% and 33% and the average length of ICU admission is 10.8 days.[4] The mortality rate among patients receiving mechanical ventilation is 43% to 67%, and it is close to 70% among patients older than 60 years.[5]

Around the world, providing safe anesthesia and critical care services has been a major challenge during the pandemic. This problem is more pronounced in LMICs. Anesthesia and critical care services are easily overwhelmed in LMICs because of the dense population with a high rate of infection, limited testing capacity and weak contact-tracing, inadequate hospital and critical care beds, inadequate anesthesiologists and intensivists, weak health care infrastructure, and limited access to therapeutics and personal protective equipment (PPE). Most LMICs responded to the COVID-19 pandemic with various public health measures, such as strict lockdown, social distancing, and universal masking. The measures were initially effective in reducing the rapid spread of the infection, but most of these stringent measures have since been relaxed in many countries. The limitations of treating critically ill patients, even in high-income countries, have been abundantly discussed in academic and public forums in the current pandemic.[6]

Epidemiology of COVID-19 in Nepal

Nepal is one of the poorest countries of the world with a nominal gross domestic product per capita of only around US$1070.[7] The first case of COVID-19 in Nepal was diagnosed in January 2020, through testing done in Hong Kong, because of the unavailability of the reverse-transcriptase polymerase chain reaction test in Nepal.[8] Because Nepal has limited health care capacity, including of intensive care beds, a strict national lockdown with social distancing measures was imposed for months, from March to July 2020. However, since easing the national lockdown, Nepal has seen a surge of COVID-19 cases and deaths.[9] As of November 8, 2020, there are more than 194,000 confirmed cases of COVID-19, with 1108 deaths in Nepal.[9] The future course and outcome of the pandemic are impossible to predict because the numbers of new infections and deaths continue to increase at an alarming rate.

DISCUSSION

The ongoing pandemic has severely affected all sectors of Nepal's health care delivery system. Anesthesia and critical care services are hard hit, because sparse health resources and public spending have been diverted to the containment of the infection, and the management of COVID-19 patients. In Nepal, the first ICU was established in 1973, and this was the only well-equipped ICU in the country for close to 20 years.[10] As of April 15, 2020, Nepal had only 1595 ICU beds for a population of nearly 30 million, and only around 850 ICU ventilators.[11] The intensive care facilities were already stretched before the pandemic, and with the rapid surge of patients requiring ICU admission, Nepal is currently experiencing a critical shortage of ICU beds.

Lately, there is a concerted effort by public and private health institutions to develop more facilities for the management of COVID-19 patients. Several existing postoperative wards and other high-dependency units have been converted into improvised critical care units. However, ICU equipment and trained personnel are scarce.[12] It is difficult to procure essential ICU equipment and personal protective devices because medical manufacturing facilities are nonexistent in the country. The government, and private institutions, have already spent enormous sums developing new makeshift ICUs and procuring consumables; it is doubtful whether most of these institutions can fund the additional cost of running optimal services in the operating rooms (ORs) and ICUs.

Early Response to the Pandemic

Nepal, like most resource-limited countries, was unprepared to face the rapid upsurge of a highly infectious disease. There was only one dedicated tertiary-level infectious disease hospital in the entire country before the current pandemic. There is also huge variability in the distribution of health care across the country, with poor health infrastructure outside a few big cities. Initially, the Government of Nepal segregated all government, and some private hospitals, into either COVID-dedicated hospital or non-COVID hospital. However, with the rapid increase in the number of patients, and limited health centers that could cater to such patients, the COVID-19 hospitals were soon overwhelmed and it was no longer possible to maintain the segregation. Currently, all hospitals in the country manage patients, irrespective of COVID-19, unless patients have to be referred to a higher center for specialized care.

After the initial lockdown, all elective surgeries were stopped as the focus shifted to managing patients with COVID-19. In many hospitals, this policy continues to date with surgical departments only treating patients with urgent or emergency conditions. With limited resources, anesthesiologists were forced to improvise to decrease the risk of contagion. Many anesthesiologists and intensivists started using videolaryngoscopes for the first time. Several types of barrier protective devices, such as transparent aerosol boxes and plastic sheets, were used to cover the patient's head during aerosol-generating procedures (eg, endotracheal intubation, airway suctioning, and extubation). Many standard recommendations that were not cost-prohibitive, such as the use of high-efficiency viral filters and minimizing aerosol-generating procedures, were followed.

CURRENT CHALLENGES TO ANESTHESIOLOGY AND CRITICAL CARE SERVICE DELIVERY IN NEPAL

The health care system in Nepal is mixed, with public health facilities and private hospitals providing health services. Public health institutions are controlled by the government and organized at central, provincial, and local levels. The infrastructure in most of the government-funded hospitals outside the large cities is weak, and often strained even at normal times.[13] Most of the ICU beds are within private health care facilities. As in many LMICs, health care facilities are concentrated in cities, but most people live in rural areas, creating inequality in access to health care. Similarly, COVID-19 testing facilities are only available in big cities. In private hospitals, surgical and intensive care costs are expensive and not readily affordable by most of the population. There are added financial constraints because the health insurance system is almost nonexistent in the country.

Infrastructure and Personnel

The capacity for critical care delivery in LMICs is limited. Most LMICs in Asia have fewer than 3 ICU beds per 100,000 population; Nepal has 2.8 ICU beds per 100,000 population, whereas Germany has 29.4 ICU beds, and the United States has 34.7 per 100,000 population.[14,15] Most of the ORs and ICUs do not have the provision of a negative-pressure system. Even in other Asian countries, less than 40% of the ICUs have the provision of negative-pressure rooms.[16] A central monitoring system and invasive and advanced monitors are limited to few tertiary-care centers.

A recent cross-sectional study of all COVID-care hospitals in Nepal found a lack of most basic equipment in the ICU.[17] Only around 63% of the hospitals had a defibrillator, and only 26.7% of hospitals could process arterial blood gas samples.[17] Nearly 47% of the hospitals did not have a central pipeline supply for oxygen. There are no published data about the availability of other essential OR and ICU equipment, such as infusion pumps, noninvasive ventilation, high-flow nasal cannula, and hospital beds equipped with oxygen supply. There is also a pressing need for more health care workers. Nepal has only 1 doctor per 1000 people, which is well lower than the World Health Organization's recommendation of 2.3 doctors per 1000 population.[18]

Most of the ICUs in the country are staffed by anesthesiologists and internists. There are few physicians with additional training in critical care. There are only a handful of critical care nurses. Other ICU workers, such as respiratory therapists and clinical pharmacists, are not found in most hospitals. Health care institutions in LMICs were already struggling with the lack of trained workers before the pandemic. With the surge of COVID-19, many health care workers have also been infected, significantly overburdening the existing hospital workforce. This may worsen outcomes for patients, because adequate staffing is crucial to maintain proper patient care.[19] Proper strategies to support and manage infected workers also seem to be lacking. In many hospitals, health care staff is now asked to work simultaneously in COVID-19 and non-COVID-19 areas of the hospital. Even infected patients have been shifted to nondesignated areas of the hospital because COVID-19-dedicated areas are overflooded with infected patients, increasing the risk of spreading the infection.

There is also a scarcity of essential anesthesia and critical care equipment for COVID-19 patients. For instance, ultrasonography and other radiologic devices may not be available in COVID-19-designated areas of the hospital. There may also be difficulty in obtaining radiographs and echocardiography tests because of the logistical difficulties in sharing the same facilities and equipment between infected and noninfected patients. This not only adds to the difficulty for the anesthesiologists and intensivists, but severely compromised patient care.

Infection Control Measures

Health care workers are at risk of contracting COVID-19 because of frequent contact with infected patients. The overall proportion of health care workers infected with COVID-19 is around 10%.[20] This proportion is approximately 18% in the United States, 4% in China, and 9% in Italy.[20] The availability of good-quality PPE kits, proper use of PPE, and infection control training programs are key to reduce the incidence of health care–associated infection. The World Health Organization has recommended the use of gloves, masks, goggles or face shields, and long-sleeved gowns with N95 respirators for aerosol-generating medical procedures. In many LMICs, the supply and availability of PPE are inadequate. The surgical masks and N95 masks are reused in most hospitals in Nepal. Because certified respirators are in short supply, the fit-test is rarely carried out. The government has encouraged local production of

PPE, but quality control and surveillance are limited, endangering the safety of health care workers. Face shields and goggles are shared after disinfection. The use of reusable elastomeric respirators and reusable powered air-purifying respirators are alternatives, but their procurement has been difficult.

An infection prevention and control (IPC) program, with a dedicated trained team at the health care facility, is recommended in all hospitals. IPC measures, if implemented appropriately, protect patients, health care workers, and visitors. In an international survey, only 11% of respondents from low-income countries had consistent access to respiratory equipment, 12% to isolation gowns, and 4% to negative-pressure rooms or personnel training in IPC.[21] Inadequate access to IPC equipment and training can lead to major COVID-19 outbreaks in hospitals and institutional isolation centers. Most hospitals in Nepal do not have the provision of IPC programs. Similarly, because of constraints of space and resources, separate areas for proper donning and doffing of PPE are not available in most ORs and ICUs, which significantly adds to the risk of viral contamination.

Quality Care

The delivery of quality care during any pandemic is challenging because crucial scientific information is always evolving. Therapeutic options may also be uncertain. A recent study found a significant disparity in the number of COVID-19-related studies and publications between high-income countries and LMICs.[21] The protocols, guidelines, and therapeutic options for COVID-19 are mostly formulated based on studies and experiences of high-income countries. However, such guidelines may not necessarily address the unique problems of resource-limited settings. Some of the standard guidelines may not even be feasible in most ORs and ICUs in Nepal and other resource-limited countries because of resource-constraints, and significant variability in the structure and composition of the workforce. Data-driven quality improvement programs in high-income countries have helped to identify gaps in health care service delivery, and design "improvement approaches." There is a glaring lack of such programs in resource-limited settings.

Future Directions

In the current pandemic, there is a significant overload of clinical information, but without the accompanying high-quality clinical research. There is a paucity of unifying clinical guidelines and a lot of uncertainty about the best treatment options, resulting in dissimilar treatment decisions between patients. There is an urgent need for research focused on LMICs, because the scientific evidence derived from high-income countries may not be accurate when applied in a different setting. For instance, the population in LMICs may be younger than in the western world and may have fewer risk factors for developing severe COVID-19, such as obesity. Most hospitals in LMICs may also not be able to meet the standards recommended by international guidelines. An option may be for international bodies to develop or propose the minimal safety standards for anesthesia and critical care services in LMICs, considering the available resources, without compromising the safety of patients and health care workers. For example, dexamethasone is readily available and can be administered in most patients. It can be prioritized over expensive therapeutics of questionable benefits that are not easily available in low-resource settings, such as newer antivirals, immunomodulators, and convalescent plasma therapy.

The current and previous pandemics have pushed innovation. These innovations are extremely handy when resources are limited. Experiences from the SARS epidemic in Hong Kong suggested that when negative-pressure isolation rooms are

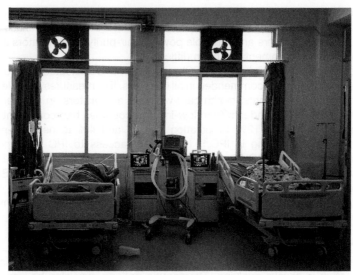

Fig. 1. Postanesthesia care unit is converted into COVID ICU. Because of lack of negative-pressure system, industrial exhaust fans were installed to minimize the viral load.

not available, normal rooms can be converted to makeshift negative-pressure rooms by the use of industrial exhaust fans.[22] In our center, we converted the postoperative care unit into a COVID ICU. We applied industrial exhaust fans over each patient bed, attempting to create negative-pressure systems and to minimize the viral load (**Fig. 1**). Similarly, several cost-effective improvised videolaryngoscopes, PPE kits, and ventilators have been designed recently.[23–27] However, these improvised surrogates should be tested for safety and effectiveness before generalized use. Because the population of the LMICs is young with possibly fewer risk factors, resource-constrained countries may still achieve acceptable clinical outcomes by determining the minimal standards of care, and doing the basics right.

SUMMARY

In resource-limited settings, it is often not possible or practicable to meet the clinical targets stipulated in international guidelines. This difficulty is more pronounced in the ongoing pandemic because the optimal use of scarce resources is crucial. It is useful for health care delivery systems in resource-limited settings to promote pragmatic innovative measures, adapt international guidelines to suit local needs, focus on diagnostic and therapeutic measures that are easily accessible and less resource-intensive, and promote native research activities. It is equally important to shift the focus beyond ICU admissions, advanced monitoring, and therapeutic requirements to other important aspects of treating COVID-19 patients where there are better chances of alleviating suffering and providing equitable care. Integrating hospice and palliative care into the health care system, which is strikingly deficient in LMICs, will also go a long way in providing dignified end-of-life care during the COVID-19 pandemic.

DISCLOSURE

The authors have nothing to disclose.

REFERENCES

1. Weiser TG, Haynes AB, Molina G, et al. Size and distribution of the global volume of surgery in 2012. Bull World Health Organ 2016;94:201–209f.
2. Alkire BC, Raykar NP, Shrime MG, et al. Global access to surgical care: a modelling study. Lancet Glob Health 2015;3e:316–23.
3. Wu Z, McGoogan JM. Characteristics of and important lessons from the coronavirus disease 2019 (COVID-19) outbreak in China: summary of a report of 72314 cases from the Chinese Center for Disease Control and Prevention. JAMA 2020; 323:1239–42.
4. Tan E, Song J, Deane AM, et al. Global impact of COVID-19 infection requiring admission to the intensive care unit: a systematic review and meta-analysis. Chest 2020;159(2):524–36.
5. Wunsch H. Mechanical ventilation in COVID-19: interpreting the current epidemiology. Am J Respir Crit Care Med 2020;202:1–4.
6. Herreros B, Gella P, Real de Asua D. Triage during the COVID-19 epidemic in Spain: better and worse ethical arguments. J Med Ethics 2020;464:55–8.
7. GDP per capita (current US$). World Bank national accounts data, and OECD National Accounts data files. Available at: https://data.worldbank.org/indicator/NY.GDP.PCAP.CD. Accessed November 1, 2020.
8. Bastola A, Sah R, Rodriguez-Morales AJ, et al. The first 2019 novel coronavirus case in Nepal. Lancet Infect Dis 2020;202:79–80.
9. Covid-19 cases map representation. Ministry of health and population Nepal. Available at: https://covid19.mohp.gov.np. Accessed November 8, 2020.
10. Acharya SP. Critical care medicine in Nepal: where are we? Int Health 2013; 59:2–5.
11. Government of Nepal: Ministry of Health and Population. Health Sector Emergency Response Plan COVID-19 Pandemic. 2020. Available at: https://www.who.int/docs/default-source/nepal-documents/novel-coronavirus/health-sector-emergency-response-plan-covid-19-endorsed-may-2020.pdf?sfvrsn=ef831f44_2. Accessed November 5, 2020.
12. Shrestha GS, Paneru HR, Acharya SP, et al. Preparedness for coronavirus disease in hospitals of Nepal: a nationwide survey. JNMA J Nepal Med Assoc 2020;582:48–51.
13. Neupane HC, Gauli B, Adhikari S, et al. Contextualizing critical care medicine in the face of COVID-19 pandemic. JNMA J Nepal Med Assoc 2020;584:47–52.
14. Phua J, Faruq MO, Kulkarni AP, et al. Critical care bed capacity in Asian countries and regions. Crit Care Med 2020;486:54–62.
15. Ma X, Vervoort D. Critical care capacity during the COVID-19 pandemic: global availability of intensive care beds. J Crit Care 2020;589:6–7.
16. Arabi YM, Phua J, Koh Y, et al. Structure, organization, and delivery of critical care in Asian ICUs. Crit Care Med 2016;44:e940–8.
17. Assessment of health-related country preparedness and readiness of Nepal for responding to COVID-19 pandemic. Preparedness and readiness of government of Nepal designated COVID hospitals 2020. Available at: http://nhrc.gov.np/wp-content/uploads/2020/06/Fact-sheet-Preparedness-and-Readiness-of-Government-of-Nepal-Designated-COVID-Hospitals.pdf. Accessed October 25, 2020.
18. The World Bank. Physicians (per 1,000 people) - Nepal. Available at: https://data.worldbank.org/indicator/SH.MED.PHYS.ZS?locations=NP. Accessed October 19, 2020.
19. Remuzzi A, Remuzzi G. COVID-19 and Italy: what next? Lancet 2020;395:1225–8.

20. Sahu AK, Amrithanand VT, Mathew R, et al. COVID-19 in health care workers: a systematic review and meta-analysis. Am J Emerg Med 2020;38:1727–31.

21. Usuzaki T, Chiba S, Shimoyama M, et al. A disparity in the number of studies related to COVID-19 and SARS-CoV-2 between low- and middle-income countries and high-income countries. Int Health 2020. https://doi.org/10.1093/inthealth/ihaa088.

22. Gomersall CD, Tai DY, Loo S, et al. Expanding ICU facilities in an epidemic: recommendations based on experience from the SARS epidemic in Hong Kong and Singapore. Intensive Care Med 2006;32:1004–13.

23. Hamal PK, Chaurasia RB, Pokhrel N, et al. An affordable videolaryngoscope for use during the COVID-19 pandemic. Lancet Glob Health 2020;8:e893–4.

24. Saoraya J, Musikatavorn K, Sereeyotin J. Low-cost videolaryngoscope in response to COVID-19 pandemic. West J Emerg Med 2020;21:817–8.

25. Chien LC, Beÿ CK, Koenig KL. A positive-pressure environment disposable shield (PEDS) for COVID-19 health care worker protection. Prehosp Disaster Med 2020;35:434–7.

26. Fang Z, Li AI, Wang H, et al. AmbuBox: a fast-deployable low-cost ventilator for COVID-19 emergent care. SLAS Technol 2020. https://doi.org/10.1177/2472630320953801. 20202472630320953801.

27. Jardim-Neto AC, Perlman CE. A low-cost off-the-shelf pressure-controlled mechanical ventilator for a mass respiratory failure scenario. Br J Anaesth 2020; 125:e438–40.

Anesthesiology in Times of Physical Disasters— Earthquakes and Typhoons

Tsui Sin Yui Cindy, MBBS[a,b,]*, Ranish Shrestha, BS[c],
Bajracharya Smriti Mahaju, MD[d], Ashish Amatya, MD[d]

KEYWORDS

- Earthquake • Typhoon • Nepal • Hong Kong • Anesthesiology • Critical care
- Emergency response • Disaster management

KEY POINTS

- Natural disasters can cause substantial damage to health care facilities and health care infrastructure.
- Earthquakes and typhoons can present with minimal advance warning, necessitating that disaster response plans are well developed and already in place before an event.
- Nepal and Hong Kong are susceptible to earthquakes and typhoons, respectively, due to their geographic locations.
- Nepal and Hong Kong have both experienced massive natural disasters in recent years, allowing their health care systems to develop comprehensive response plans.

INTRODUCTION

Physical disasters occur worldwide, in different forms, and may cause widespread traumatic injury and death. Anesthesiologists, through their work in both the surgical and intensive care settings, may provide critical services in the aftermath of natural disasters. Earthquakes and typhoons are 2 of the most common physical disasters that may lead to widespread destruction, both human and environmental. This article explores the role of anesthesia specialists in the medical response to physical disasters, using the recent earthquake in Nepal and the frequent encounters with typhoons in Hone Kong (HK) as case studies.

[a] Department of Anaesthesia and Intensive Care, The Chinese University of Hong Kong, 30-32 Ngan Shing Street, Shatin New Territories 852, Hong Kong; [b] Prince of Wales Hospital, 30-32 Ngan Shing Street, Shatin New Territories 852, Hong Kong; [c] Infection Control Unit, Nepal Cancer Hospital and Research Center, Harisiddhi-28, Lalitpur 44700, Nepal; [d] Department of Cardiac Anaesthesiology and Critical Care, Shahid Gangalal National Heart Center, P.O. Box-11360, Kathmandu 44600, Nepal
* Corresponding author. Prince of Wales Hospital, 30-32 Ngan Shing Street, Shatin New Territories 852, Hong Kong.
E-mail address: cindytsui@cuhk.edu.hk

Anesthesiology Clin 39 (2021) 293–308
https://doi.org/10.1016/j.anclin.2021.02.005
1932-2275/21/© 2021 Elsevier Inc. All rights reserved.

anesthesiology.theclinics.com

EARTHQUAKES

The World Health Organization defines an earthquake as the "violent and abrupt shaking of the ground, caused by movement between tectonic plates along a fault line in the earth's crust... [and]... can result in the ground shaking, soil liquefaction, landslides, fissures, avalanches, fires and tsunamis."[1] In a report compiling the cumulative losses by various natural disasters between 1998 and 2017, approximately 125 million people are estimated to have been affected by earthquakes through injuries, homelessness, displacement, or other economic losses, with earthquakes accounting for 56% (747,234) of all deaths and 23% ($661 billion) of economic losses due to such disasters.[2] Mortality and morbidity are the immediate effects of earthquakes, which are exacerbated by disruption of essential services, such as sanitation, infrastructure, and health care facilities.[3] Consequently, diarrhea, skin, and respiratory infections are to be anticipated.[4]

The Role of the Anesthesiologist in the Event of an Earthquake

The primary cause of mortality and trauma during earthquakes is the collapse of physical structures.[5] The day-to-day role of an anesthesiologist routinely involves resuscitation, perioperative management, critical care, and pain management. All of these skills are essential in the management of trauma patients during an earthquake, especially in providing first aid, performing preoperative and postoperative resuscitation, rehabilitation, and pain management.[6] Anesthesiologists learn disaster management skills throughout their training, so they are competent in providing treatment to people injured in earthquakes.

Prehospital Care

Earthquakes may produce severe blunt trauma with crush injuries, wound infections, and burns and often require multiple surgical procedures.[7,8] Victims of earthquakes who can be saved are not those who are killed by fatal wounds to the head and chest due to dismantling structures but those with injuries that may cause mortality over several hours, for example, by manageable conditions, such as slow exsanguination. Thus, early treatment determines the prognosis for earthquake victims.[9] More lives may be saved if the time from injury to treatment can be minimized by providing prompt and effective triage and treatment.

The role of surgery and anesthesia is particularly important, therefore, within the first 24 hours to 48 hours after an earthquake and may include resuscitation of patients in the field, airway management, and establishing vascular access for hemodynamic stabilization and transport to a hospital.

Due to frequent damage to infrastructure, earthquakes often are characterized by the need for critical care in the field, limited supplies and medical personnel, and the need to establish triage protocols to prioritize patient transport to more definitive medical facilities. In such conditions, anesthesiologists may be designated as "trauma anesthesia/critical care specialists" and function as team leaders in the prehospital period in some parts of the world.[10] Several studies have shown prehospital tracheal intubation of severely injured patients to be potentially unsafe if delivered without appropriate drugs, monitoring, equipment, training, and clinical guidance.[11–14] Utilizing anesthesiologists in prehospital care can lead to a survival benefit.[15–19]

In-hospital Care

Traumatic injuries frequently require surgical intervention, and intraoperative anesthetic technique is important to optimize patient outcomes. In a mass casualty disaster, such as an earthquake, the priority is choosing an anesthetic technique that facilitates early recovery and discharge from the hospital, thereby allowing care to be provided to a high volume of patients. The choice of anesthesia depends on a patient's characteristics and surgical procedure and most importantly available resources.[20]

Type of Anesthesia

Regarding the type of anesthesia to be used, 2 guiding principles are recommended: (1) cardiorespiratory depression and muscular relaxation should be avoided, and (2) dependence on oxygen or electronic monitoring should be reduced. Epidural anesthesia is not recommended and inhalational anesthetics have limitations.[21] General anesthesia may not be available in many hospitals in disaster areas.[22] Among various types of anesthesia, regional anesthesia has been highly encouraged and widely used, with good results during emergencies in resource-poor conditions,[23] in both civilian and military settings, and has been reported to be a valuable tool following several natural disasters.[24–26]

Regional anesthesia is associated with fewer side effects, greater hemodynamic stability, a high success rate, and low electrical power requirements.[27] During the earthquake in Haiti in 2010, many patients received regional anesthesia using ultrasound-guided regional nerve blocks (from lumbar plexus block to sciatic block).[22] A study by Missair and colleagues[28] reports the use of femoral/sciatic nerve blocks as well as axillary and interscalene nerve blocks without any perioperative anesthesia complications or pain, with a success rate of approximately 90%.

Because regional anesthesia often uses and ultrasound facility, that might be a limitation during disaster conditions.[20] During an earthquake, electronic monitoring systems may be compromised due to lack of electricity, thus requiring the anesthesia team to monitor the patient manually.[21] During the Haiti earthquake, only manual blood pressure and pulse oximetry were used as monitors.[22]

Anesthetic Agent

In disaster areas, ketamine may be particularly useful as an intravenous anesthetic agent.[29,30] Ketamine has a favorable safety profile from cardiovascular and respiratory perspectives, especially in disaster settings where hemorrhagic shock is a concern. It increases blood pressure and heart rate with preservation of airway reflexes. In addition, it provides both analgesia and anesthesia. Hence, ketamine is listed as a World Health Organization (WHO) essential medication. During the 2005 Kashmir earthquake, one team reported that they intervened in 180 surgical patients; they used general anesthesia in 44% of the patients and also used ketamine 41% of the time. They stated that ketamine is a safe and sufficient agent for anesthesia for surgical procedures performed in the field due to the lack of complications and good surgeon satisfaction.[29,31]

Postoperative Analgesia

Adequate pain control is critical for the successful recovery of trauma patients following surgery and is a skill set with which anesthesiologists are well versed. It is well known that inadequate acute pain control can lead to the development of chronic pain. Approximately 80% of the global population lives in areas where access to pain medication is inadequate,[32,33] and prioritizing pain control often is neglected after disasters.

History of Anesthesiology in Nepal

When the 1934 earthquake struck Nepal, Bir Hospital was the only hospital. There were no other hospitals or qualified anesthesiologists to manage trauma victims during that time. There is no evidence of anesthesia practice in Nepal prior to 1933. In those days, anesthesia services were provided by any experienced medical or paramedical staff by pouring chloroform or ether onto a Schimmelbusch mask.[34] By 1984, there were 7 qualified anesthesiologists in Nepal who were trained outside of the country. In 1985, a 1-year diploma in anesthesia program was started by the Institute of Medicine teaching hospital.[35] The country has evolved from having no trained anesthesiologists during the 1930s, to having 7 qualified anesthesiologists between 1955 and 1984, to more than 300 registered anesthesiologists currently.[36]

Earthquakes in the Context of Nepal

Nepal ranks eleventh among the most earthquake-prone nations.[37] The Himalayan arc (containing the youngest mountain peaks in the world) were formed by the collision of the Indian plate into the Eurasian plate, which still is an ongoing process.[38] Approximately one-third of the length of the Himalayas lies within Nepal; thus, Nepal lies in a highly active seismic vault between the 2 plates. Based on the seismic activity, it is expected that an earthquake of magnitude greater than 8 on the Richter scale would occur every 130 years to 260 years. The last such earthquake occurred on January 15, 1934 (Nepal–Bihar earthquake), and caused significant damage to the Kathmandu Valley and surrounding areas.[39]

The 2015 Earthquake

An earthquake measuring 7.8 on the Richter scale struck Nepal on April 25, 2015, with the epicenter being the Barpak region of Gorkha District, 80 km northwest of the Kathmandu Valley. The Kathmandu Valley, along with Nuwakot, Rasuwa, Sindhupalchok, Dhading, and Gorkha, were the hardest hit districts. This was followed by a second earthquake (Richter scale 7.3), 17 days later. Of the 75 districts, 31 were affected, of which 14 were prioritized for rescue, relief, and recovery operations.[40] The earthquake claimed 8896 lives; injured 22,302; and displaced 649,815 families; and approximately 893,786 private houses were fully or partially destroyed, causing total damage and loss valued at $7 billion.

Most of the injuries were concentrated in the Kathmandu Valley,[41] with more than 30% of all primary health centers and 46% of all hospitals in the 14 most affected districts fully or partially damaged.[42] Due to dramatic variability of Nepal's physical geography, Nepal's health care system already was strained before the earthquake. In remote areas, only primary-level health care posts are available, which are supervised by health either or medical assistants and rarely by medical doctors. Because transportation is difficult and ambulances cannot reach, even in normal times, the earthquake exaggerated shortages of essential emergency drugs, oxygen supply, and basic medical needs.[43]

The health care sector was hit especially hard, with 446 public health centers completely destroyed.[44] The earthquake, however, did not cause much damage to the health centers and hospitals within the Kathmandu Valley,[21] including Kathmandu's largest public hospitals, including Tribhuvan University Teaching Hospital (TUTH), Patan Hospital, Civil Service Hospital, Birendra Army Hospital, and the trauma center at Bir Hospital, largely due to the retrofitting done in anticipation of such an event.[45]

Government-Level Response to the Earthquake

The Natural Calamity Relief Act has provisions to set up different institutions to administer relief and rescue work during an emergency. The Central Natural Disaster Relief Committee (CNDRC), within the Home Ministry, is the apex body of disaster management in Nepal. Disaster management in Nepal is mostly relief and response focused.[37] The National Emergency Operation Center, under the CNDRC, was activated at level IV disaster under the National Disaster Response Framework. The Home Secretary led the central command, and search and rescue were conducted by security forces.[41]

Nepal's Ministry of Health and Population (MoHP), with the medical command center of the Nepalese Army, was one of the facilitators of the response within the health sector. The MoHP activated the Health Emergency Operations Center to coordinate and provide emergency medical teams (EMTs) to various affected regions of the country, along with allocation of the Nepal Police and Armed Police Force.[43]

Nepal experienced an overwhelming international response following the earthquake in 2015. Within the first few hours after the earthquake, the Nepalese government issued a statement calling for international support, which translated into assistance from 36 nations.[46] Teams from India and Bangladesh arrived within 12 hours, followed by China, Sri Lanka, and other Southeast Asian Nations. Several humanitarian organizations, including the United Nations, Doctors Without Borders, International Committee of the Red Cross, International Federation of Red Cross and Red Crescent Societies, Oxfam, CARE International, International Medical Corps, and Save the Children all provided assistance. The cluster of UN agencies was coordinated by the World Food Program.[47] The World Food Program coordinated the storage and movement of relief materials.

International EMTs from 127 organizations and 36 nations provided medical services, allowing provision of 8697 outpatient consultations, 486 inpatient beds, and 91 surgeries per day. As elaborated by Cook and colleagues,[46] the immediate relief phase focused on 4 key areas: (1) strategic planning, (2) aid delivery, (3) aid provision, and (4) aid distribution. Of the people affected by the earthquake, approximately 117,000 were treated in outpatient departments; 41,200 were hospitalized; and a total of 7124 surgical operations (including 41 amputations) were performed within 2 weeks.[42] Most of the injuries were musculoskeletal in nature. At Om hospital, a private hospital in Kathmandu, 1900 cases were managed in the emergency department within the first 3 days of the earthquake, of which 80 underwent musculoskeletal surgery.[40] The active participation of anesthesiologists saved the lives of many seriously injured earthquake victims.

At TUTH, one of the major tertiary centers in Kathmandu, critical care capacity was limited on the day of the earthquake, with only 11 level 3 intensive care unit (ICU) beds and 10 level 2 beds equipped with advanced monitoring. Within the first few hours of the earthquake, the critical care capacity within the hospital was doubled, whereas within the first week, 478 major procedures were performed.[49] The triage area was modified by dividing the red zone into an acute resuscitation area and space for preoperative assessment for those requiring immediate surgery; 1812 patients were managed in the emergency department, whereas 591 underwent major surgery.[50]

Like in most developing countries, including Nepal, ICU patients are managed by anesthesiologists. Critical care services, which are not fully established throughout Nepal, were overwhelmed due to severe shortages of basic needs, such as essential drugs, surgical gowns, gloves, hand sanitizers, and oxygen needed to care for people with life-threatening illnesses.[51] Due to trauma victims from the earthquake filling up ICU beds, patients with other serious illnesses were displaced. These circumstances forced early discharges from hospitals, which eventually resulted in readmissions and likely preventable deaths.[49]

At Dhulikhel Hospital, a university hospital east of Kathmandu, a total of 1083 earthquake-related injuries were treated—58% were fractures—and a total of 345 surgical procedures were performed.[52] The experience of a field hospital established by the Israeli Defense Forces that treated more than 1600 patients, with more than 100 surgeries within 11 days documents the use of regional anesthesia.[53] Of orthopedic and plastic surgery procedures, 96% were conducted using regional nerve blocks, either a femoral or saphenous block, a high or low sciatic block, or a combination. Interscalene or supraclavicular blocks were used for hand, arm, and shoulder surgery. The report documents the benefits of regional anesthesia, which, in addition to those discussed previously, included reduced requirement for postoperative opioid use. Likewise, use of regional anesthesia allowed for quick patient mobilization and evacuation in case of aftershocks. Intravenous ketamine (along with midazolam) was used for mild sedation.[53]

Challenges

One of the major issues after the earthquake was the lack of adequate space for international relief-bearing air carriers at the Tribhuwan International Airport, which acted as a chokepoint, causing many international teams to be delayed for days or to be rerouted to Calcutta or Dhaka. The difficult terrain and roads, obstructed by landslides, impaired relief and rescue beyond Kathmandu, allowing only small aircraft to be mobilized in such areas. Also, communication challenges between civil aviation and rescue operations led to miscommunication and almost led to midair collisions in the Nepali airspace.[46]

Poor coordination between the national and local government,[54] UN bodies, nongovernmental organizations, international nongovernmental organizations, and foreign military delayed relief distribution and created confusion, resulting in some regions receiving multiple response teams whereas others received none.[37] A gap between the required relief materials (shelters, tents, and so forth) and what was available was not met by the relief delivery.[41]

One of the primary limitations of regional anesthesia was the language barrier between the patients and international EMTs, impeding communication.[53] Lack of equipment and skilled human resources to perform complex procedures were some of the challenges faced. Medical supplies, such as implants, were in short supply.[48] The situation was exacerbated by the 4-month border closure between India and Nepal, which resulted in a shortage of medications and fuel, thus further limiting health service provision.[55]

TYPHOONS

A typhoon is an ocean storm—a rapidly rotating cyclone associated with heavy rains. It commonly affects costal countries and islands during the hot and humid summer. Depending on the site of origin, sometimes it is called a hurricane or tropical cyclone. Typhoon damage is proportional to its strength. Its damage could be related to a direct effect (such as flooding and storm surge) or indirect effects (such as landslides and wind-related flying objects). Escalated demands for anesthesia and critical care services during typhoons normally are sustained over days. A thorough framework is needed to enable all parties to be fully informed and respond effectively, and risk management and contingency plans involve strategies for management throughout from pretyphoon through the recovery period.

What Makes Typhoons Happen?

A typhoon is an ocean storm—a rapidly rotating cyclone associated with heavy rains.[56] When the wind speed intensifies to 118 km per hour in the Northwest Pacific, it is called a typhoon. When it originates in the North Atlantic, central North Pacific, and eastern North Pacific, the term hurricane is used. Meanwhile, in the South Pacific and Indian Ocean, the term, tropical cyclone, is used, regardless of its strength.[57] Typhoons often take unpredictable loops.[58]

Typhoons are generated over warm ocean waters during the summer. As the wind passes over the ocean's surface, water evaporates. Water vapor cools on rising and condense into water droplets, forming large clouds. Heat in the vapor is released to the surrounding air. Air at the top becomes warmer and elevates air pressure causing winds to move outward. As the evaporation process continues, there is constant rising of moisture, which creates a low-pressure area at the surface. Air pushes into this low-pressure area. The "new" air becomes warm and rises too. With this continuous heated moisture from the warm ocean as the fuel, the whole system of clouds and wind spins. When the wind speed is sufficiently high, it becomes a typhoon. Typhoons usually weaken when they hit land because they no longer are fed by the warm ocean moisture. The cloud system, however, may start dumping many inches of rain.[59] Tropical storms are are encountered in the South China Sea.[60,61] On average, HK witnesses 6 typhoons per year.[6] As such, HK tops Asia's rankings as the city with the greatest natural disaster risk within a highly urbanized community and population density.[62]

Destructive Power of a Typhoon

The damage inflicted by a typhoon is proportional to its strength. In HK, since 2009, any storm with wind speeds more than 185 km per hour at its center is categorized as a super-typhoon. A storm with 150 km to 184 km per hour maximum wind at the center is a severe typhoon.[63] Typhoons may cause an array of damage, both direct and indirect.[64]

Direct Damage: Flooding and Storm Surge

Devastating floods result from squally showers. In mountainous terrain, water runoff accumulates in restricted valleys and flows downstream in a huge flooding wave. It concentrates sediment and debris.[64] Together with strong on-shore wind, it causes a rise in sea level that leads to severe inundation of coastal areas. This storm surge is aggravated further by high tides. When this occurs, loss of life could be due to drowning, either from the rise in sea water inundating the land or from floods. Seafaring livelihoods are exposed because large boats may be washed around in outlying islands.[65]

Indirect Damage: Landslides, Flying Objects, and Heat Waves

Damage may occur with heavy rain, even in the absence of severe wind. Landslides cause significant destructive damage. Households situated near slopes and loose soils are affected the most. Structural glazing and inclusion of balconies are common nowadays, and flying objects from these, as well as unauthorized building projects, may cause wind-related injuries (**Figs. 1** and **2**). Typhoons knock down trees and injure people when they fall. If they fall over roadways, they may lead to road traffic accidents. Fallen items also require resources and time for removal.[65] The subsiding air ahead of the typhoon is accompanied by heat waves. The heat can trigger exhaustion and exacerbate chronic illness in susceptible patients.[66]

HK has been hit by super-typhoons Hato and Mangkhut. Despite advancements in wind protection, there still were more than 60,000 reports of fallen trees, 500 reports of smashed windows, and a tower crane blown down, resulting in rooftop homes

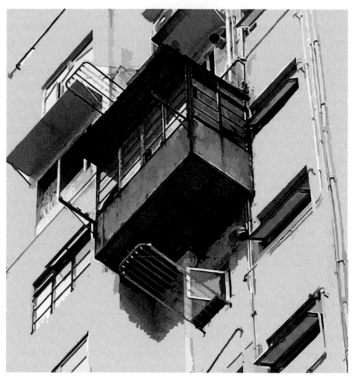

Fig. 1. An example of unauthorized building work, which commonly occurs in densely populated areas.

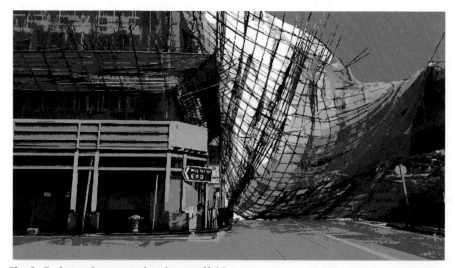

Fig. 2. Typhoon damage to bamboo scaffold.

collapsed during Mangkhut.[67] Severe flooding by storm surge submerged underground apartments, and hundreds of vessels were stranded.

Clinical Challenges During Typhoons

A typhoon is considered a slow-onset, anticipated disaster, because the prewarning signal usually comes at least a few hours before its arrival. When Mangkhut passed through HK, 458 injuries were noted.[68] It also had a severe impact on health care delivery. The electric supply was interrupted for more than 24 hours, and the supply of fresh water was affected due to power outages. Medical facilities also were affected.[67] Sea, land, and air transportation services were paralyzed. Owing to fallen trees and flooding, major roads were closed and public transportation could not be resumed for days. Regional hospital transfer of patients to tertiary centers was impacted by toppled trees and winds,[69] and patients with medical needs had to be stabilized in outlying islands because helipads were damaged. Failed meal deliveries to hospitals without kitchens were also noted.[69] Within the hospital, the shaking of doors triggered alarms in the operating theaters (OTs) and ICUs, causing unnecessary nuisance and concern.

Preparedness and Response in Anesthesia and Critical Care During a Typhoon

Escalated demand for anesthesia and critical care services during a typhoon normally is sustained over days. Yet, resource limitations also may last for days due to staff transportation breakdown, power interruption, and supply shortages. Hence, all OT and ICU staff should prepare to receive and stabilize patients with a variety of subspecialized needs (eg, obesity and trauma) in the first 48 hours.[70]

Action framework for anesthesia and intensive care during a typhoon
Pretyphoon period. Regular inspection of structural glazing and the ceiling system in the ICU and OT is important. These structures must withstand the forces of a typhoon. During hospital planning, sophisticated monitoring and response continuity plans by gas and power suppliers should be incorporated. Backup power supply and voltage stabilization could be used to prepare for any network interruption. The most sensitive systems affected are the air conditioning and escalator lifts.[71] Hence, additional venting should be in place to prepare for power outages. Cable inspection should be held regularly, with more frequent inspection during typhoon season. Flood gates could be built at the hospital entrance. Hospital transmission lines that are vulnerable to damage should be identified with contingency commuting plans. Trees should be stabilized to reduce the risk of collapse.

Stock assessment for consumables and limited resources like blood, anesthetics, ventilators, and personal protective equipment, should be carried out on a regular basis, and backup access should be procured. To ensure smooth workflow, platforms need to be strengthened to access electronic medical records and location tracking of high-risk patients. Telemedicine systems could assist with critical care triage.

There should be a well-defined level of response system in place within the hospital system. When there is an impending storm, there should be an alert issued through an information services platform to the media and emergency response center. The contingency plan would include scalable resources supported by transportation agencies to ramp up staffing and cars for potential breakdowns in commuter traffic. This would enable medical personnel to report to duty. Individual units also may arrange for shuttle bus service.

Due consideration should be given to the prevailing situations faced by individual staff members. Priority should be given to employees with special needs, such as pregnancy.[72] Because staff may be required to work beyond their normal shifts, provision of sufficient rest breaks and overnight facilities are vital. Safety facilities, such as helmets and communication devices, are essential for staff involved in patients' transfer outdoors.[72]

Well-developed contingency plans, coordinated by a disaster control center, are required to enable all parties to be fully informed and respond effectively.[73] There usually is a critical care expert to optimize surge capacity planning. The center would closely monitor road conditions, patient data, and bed and surgical capacity. Timely provision of incident updates to hospitals allows a facility to tailor its response to the demands of the incident.

Within the cluster area, a mechanism should be in place to keep essential personnel appraised of critical care resources and specific needs. Surgical and critical care resources would be developed and anticipated based on regional risks.[74] **Table 1** shows how the patient surge capacity may be managed. Because there always are resource limitations, efforts also should be made to reduce use of critical resources. For example, when an impending typhoon alert is issued, patients on oxygen should be given contingency plans for the loss of central oxygen. The identification of patients with impending needs and transportation of them to appropriate facilities early for stabilization are highly beneficial.

All staff should understand how their hospital participates in the response process. Staff could participate in regular interagency orientation as well as drills to be familiar with the skills they will need to fulfill their roles in a disaster response.[73] Useful training for ICU and OT staff should include crisis management, initial resuscitation for special needs patients, and communication. Experienced staff could receive triage training to ensure resource stewardship.[73] Staff should be provided with plans about evacuation routes, safety shelters, and backup resources.[72] Staff should have accurate information to assist patients regarding when and where to seek care and other available resources.

Super-typhoon period. When a severe typhoon is about to arrive, consideration should be given to delaying elective surgical cases. Patients already undergoing surgery will need continued care. Otherwise, all other elective services should be postponed. If the demand for emergency anesthesia and ICU services exceeds the normal capacity, contingency plans may be activated. Depending on transfer options and feasibility, patients could be diverted to other units for care.

Only essential anesthesia and critical care staff would remain on duty until the next shift of staff arrives. Essential staff usually includes those who need to continue with

Table 1
Surge capacity: mechanisms to increase patient care capacity in the event additional locations and resources are needed due to increased patient volume

Targets	Surge Capacity	Strategies
Conventional care	20% beyond usual capacity	Using resources immediately available[75] • Opening an additional emergency department • Discharging patient to lower-intensity care beds • Opening up vacant beds in the ICU
Contingency care	100% beyond usual capacity	Typically requires care to be provided in nontraditional areas[76] • Using OT areas as ICUs • Preplanning with supplemental equipment (monitors, beds, ventilators) • Anesthesia machines employed as ICU ventilators

emergency anesthesia, intensive care, and resuscitation. To avoid interruption, these staff should report to their supervisors upon arrival. Careful selection of shuttle bus pickup points with sufficient capacity is essential. All cars should be parked in sheltered areas. Staff anticipating that they would have difficulty traveling should consider staying in the hospital resting area. It is expected the major public transport systems may cease with short notice.[72]

All other staff are to remain available at home because extra staff may be required depending on occupancy and complexity. Coordination typically is through their supervisors who communicate regularly with the control center. In case of supervisors not contactable, the next most senior staff on the floor should assume control. The most common medical needs encountered during a typhoon are related to chronic illness. Relatively minor trauma, in diabetes, for example, could lead to complicated infections. Hence, exhaustive efforts to improve access to pharmaceuticals is essential.[77]

When a major disaster situation occurs, setting up a mini–control station could centralize understanding of resource availability and contact information. Nurse managers could update clinicians regularly. If the situation warrants, a resuscitation team may be needed at the site of the incident. Providing timely information on appropriate locations for people to seek care will allow for greater efficiency in screening and treating patients. It is the supervisor's decision to activate group paging, radiobroadcasting, or have police go door to door for calling in additional medical staff support. If a facility is hit by hurricane-force winds, all internal doors should be kept tightly shut, and windows should be secured with bars and any temporary structures should be secured. Gutters and storm drains should be cleared of leaves and rubbish.[71] Staff should ensure patients in the ICU are located away from glass windows on the exposed side, because they are prone to shatter.[72]

Recovery period. In the aftermath of a typhoon or other natural disaster, orderly de-escalation of resources is important. Usually there is a rebound in elective surgeries after a typhoon,[74] and decisions need to be made about which services should be provided based on a consideration of

1. Consequences of further delays in surgery
2. Resource requirements
3. Ability to provide the resources immediately following the typhoon

Patients should be notified early and kept appraised of developments to give them an idea when they could safely return to the hospital for elective surgery.

During Mangkhut, there were multiple fallen trees obstructing the entrances of the hospital, leaving tree trimming teams a massive workload.[78] In terms of repairs, priority should be given to major road ways to the hospital, thereby improving access of emergency vehicles as well as patients seeking medical care for less severe issues. Individual hospitals may need to deploy teams to provide temporary pumping facilities and alleviate any flood damage. All temporary electric facilities should be checked to ensure proper function. There often is an investigation to evaluate any deaths, injuries, or property damage after a large typhoon.

FUTURE DIRECTION

As a result of global warming, the number of intense tropical cyclones and the associated health care demands will increase. Sea level rise, secondary to global warming, also will raise the threat of storm surge. Clinical care during a typhoon requires teamwork and planning. Efforts should be made to constantly strive to learn from previous experiences, update contingency plans, and develop new ways to provide the safest and most efficient care for patients in times of natural disaster.

DISCLOSURE

The authors have nothing to disclose.

REFERENCES

1. World Health Organization. Earthquakes. 2020. Available at: https://www.who.int/health-topics/earthquakes. Accessed August 10, 2020.
2. UNISDR and CRED (United Nations Office for Disaster Risk Reduction/Center for Research on the Epidemiology of Disasters). Economic Losses, Poverty & Disasters: 1998–2017. 2018. Available at: https://www.preventionweb.net/publications/view/61119. Accessed August 7, 2020.
3. Gutiérrez E, Taucer F, De Groeve T, et al. Analysis of worldwide earthquake mortality using multivariate demographic and seismic data. Am J Epidemiol 2005; 161(12):1151–8.
4. Auerbach P. Preparedness explains some differences between Haiti and Nepal's response to earthquake. BMJ 2015;350(jun05 1):h3059.
5. Noji E. The public health consequences of disasters. Oxford University Press; 1997.
6. Filipescu Z. Problems of anesthesia and resuscitation of the victims of the bulgarian earthquake. Disaster Med 1980;245–7.
7. Missair A, Pretto E, Visan A, et al. A Matter of Life or Limb? A Review of Traumatic Injury Patterns and Anesthesia Techniques for Disaster Relief After Major Earthquakes. Anesth Analg 2013;117(4):934–41.
8. Fan Z, Li A, Lian B, et al. Injury types of victims in the 12th May 2008 Wenchuan earthquake: analysis of 1,038 patients in Jiangyou City. Eur J Trauma Emerg Surg 2010;37(1):3–7.
9. Schultz C, Koenig K, Noji E. A Medical Disaster Response to Reduce Immediate Mortality after an Earthquake. NEJM 1996;334(7):438–44.
10. Grande C, Baskett P, Donchin Y, et al. Trauma Anethesia for Disasters. Crit Care Clin 1991;7(2):339–61.
11. Davis D, Hoyt D, Ochs M, et al. The Effect of Paramedic Rapid Sequence Intubation on Outcome in Patients with Severe Traumatic Brain Injury. J Trauma Inj Infect Crit Care 2003;54(3):444–53.
12. Wang HE, Peitzman AB, Cassidy LD, et al. Out-of-hospital endotracheal intubation and outcome after traumatic brain injury. Ann Emerg Med 2004;44:439–53.
13. Murray JA, Demetriades D, Berne TV, et al. Prehospital intubation in patients with severe head injury. J Trauma Inj Infect Crit Care 2000;49:1065–70.
14. Lockey D, Davies G, Coats T. Survival of trauma patients who have prehospital tracheal intubation without anaesthesia or muscle relaxants: observational study. BMJ 2001;323:141.
15. Baxt WG, Moody P. The impact of a physician as part of the aeromedical prehospital team in patients with blunt trauma. JAMA 1987;257:3246–50.
16. Berlot G, La Fata C, Bacer B, et al. Influence of prehospital treatment on the outcome of patients with severe blunt traumatic brain injury: a single-centre study. Eur J Emerg Med 2009;16:312–7.

17. Eich C, Roessler M, Nemeth M, et al. Characteristics and outcome of prehospital paediatric tracheal intubation attended by anaesthesia-trained emergency physicians. Resuscitation 2009;80:1371–7.
18. Abbott D, Brauer K, Hutton K, et al. Aggressive out-of-hospital treatment regimen for severe closed head injury in patients undergoing air medical transport. Air Med J 1998;17:94–100.
19. Klemen P, Grmec S. Effect of pre-hospital advanced life support with rapid sequence intubation on outcome of severe traumatic brain injury. Acta Anaesthesiol Scand 2006;50:1250–4.
20. Sumartono CS, Sulistiawan SS, Semedi BP, et al. The role of anesthesiologist and selection of effective anesthesia techniques in lombok's earthquake victim's management. Preprints 2020;2020020377.
21. Centurion MT, Van Den Bergh R, Gray H. Anesthesia provision in disasters and armed conflicts. Curr Anesthesiology Rep 2017;7(1):1–7.
22. Osteen KD. Orthopedic anesthesia in Haiti. Ochsner J 2011;11(1):12–3.
23. Morey TE, Rice MJ. Anesthesia in an austere setting: lessons learned from the Haiti relief operation. Anesthesiol Clin 2013;31:107–15.
24. Bartels SA, VanRooyen MJ. Medical complications associated with earthquakes. Lancet 2012;379:748–57.
25. Bar-On E, Abargel A, Peleg K, et al. Coping with the challenges of early disaster response: 24 years of field hospital experience after earthquakes. Disaster Med Public Health Preparedness 2013;7:491–8.
26. Chen G, Lai W, Liu F, et al. The dragon strikes: lessons from the Wenchuan earthquake. Anesth Analg 2010;110:908–15.
27. Buckenmaier CC III, Lee EH, Shields CH, et al. Regional anesthesia in austere environments. Reg Anesth pain Med 2003;28(4):321–7.
28. Missair A, Gebhard R, Pierre E, et al. Surgery under extreme conditions in the aftermath of the 2010 Haiti earthquake: the importance of regional anesthesia. Prehosp Disaster Med 2010;25(6):487–93.
29. Mulvey J, Qadri A. Maqsood. Earthquake injuries and the use of ketamine for surgical procedures: the Kashmir experience. Anaesth Intensive Care 2006;34: 489–94.
30. Svenson J, Abernathy M. Ketamine for prehospital use: new look at an old drug. Am J Emerg Med 2007;25:977–80.
31. Ashraf M, Sheikh IA, Ullah Waleem SS. Anaesthetic Management ofMass Casualties-What Should Be the Drug of Choice? Pakistan *Armed Forces Med J* 2006;56:390–3.
32. World Health Organization. Postoperative care 2020. Available at: https://www.who.int/surgery/publications/Postoperativecare.pdf. Accessed September 5, 2020.
33. Goucke CR, Chaudakshetrin P. Pain: a neglected problem in the low-resource setting. Anesth Analg 2018;126(4):1283–6.
34. Amatya R. Evolution of Anesthesia in Nepal: A historical perspective. J Soc Anesthesiologists Nepal 2014;1(1):3–6.
35. Shrestha BM, Rana NB. Training and development of anesthesia in Nepal-1985 to 2005. Can J Anaesth 2006;53(4):339–43.
36. Nepal LP. Anesthesia in Nepal: From history to current scenario. Anaesth Pain Intensive Care 2019;23(1):102–4.
37. Koirala P, Jayasawal R. Emerging trends in disaster management policy in Nepal. Nepal Disaster Rep 2015;79–91.
38. Dmowska R. Advances in geophysics. Elsevier; 2003.

39. Pandey MR, Tandukar RP, Avouac JP, et al. Seismotectonics of the Nepal Himalaya from a local seismic network. J Asian Earth Sci 1999;17(5–6):703–12.

40. Government of Nepal, National Planning Commission. Nepal earthquake 2015, post disaster needs assessment. Vol. A: key Findings. Kathmandu: Government of Nepal, National Planning Commission; 2015. Available at: http://npc.gov.np/images/category/PDNA_Volume_A.pdf. Accessed September 7, 2020.

41. Government of Nepal. Ministry of home Affairs (MoHA) and disaster preparedness network-Nepal (DPNet-Nepal). Disaster report 2015. Kathmandu (Nepal): The Government of Nepal, Ministry of Home Affairs (MoHA) and Disaster Preparedness Network-Nepal (DPNet-Nepal); 2015. Available at: http://drrportal.gov.np/uploads/document/329.pdf. Web. Accessed September 7, 2020.

42. Government of Nepal, Ministry of Health and Population, HEOC. Health sector response situation update report earthquake 2015. Kathmandu (Nepal): Ministry of Health and Population, Government of Nepal; 2015. Available at: http://heoc.mohp.gov.np/attachments/article/73/02_June_2015_sit_update_HEOC.pdf. Accessed April 25, 2020.

43. Camacho NA, Karki K, Subedi S, et al. International emergency medical teams in the aftermath of the 2015 Nepal Earthquake. Prehosp Disaster Med 2019;34(3):260–4.

44. Molden D, Sharma E, Acharya G. Lessons from Nepal's Gorkha earthquake 2015. Lessons from Nepal's earthquake for the Indian Himalayas and the Gangetic plains. Kathmandu (Nepal): ICIMOD; 2016. Available at: https://www.flagship2.nrrc.org.np/sites/default/files/knowledge/Lessons%20from%20the%20Nepal%20Ghorka%202015%20Earthquake%20-%20ICIMOD%20.pdf. Accessed September 28, 2020.

45. World Health Organization. Emergency preparedness pays off as Kathmandu hospitals respond to earthquakes 2015. Available at: https://www.who.int/news-room/detail/13-05-2015-emergency-preparedness-pays-off-as-kathmandu-hospitals-respond-to-earthquakes. Accessed October 1, 2020.

46. Cook AD, Shrestha M, Htet ZB. International response to 2015 Nepal earthquake lessons and observations. Centre for Non Traditional Security Studies (NTS), S. Rajaratnam School of International Studies; 2016.

47. De Annuntiis V. Humanitarian Civil-Military Coordination in the Nepal Earthquake Response. (presented at the Regional Consultative Group on Humanitarian Civil-Military Coordination for Asia and the Pacific, Bangkok, Thailand, December 3–4, 2015).

48. Vaishya R, Agarwal AK, Vijay V, et al. Surgical management of musculoskeletal injuries after 2015 Nepal earthquake: our experience. Cureus 2015;7(8):e306.

49. Aryal D, Acharya SP, Shrestha GS, et al. Nepal after the disaster. Insider points of view for the future of critical care medicine. Am J Respir Crit Care Med 2015;192(7):781–4.

50. Bista NR. From no anesthesiologist to qualified anaesthesiologists for devastating earthquake. Abstract from 9th International Symposium on History of Anesthesia (2017), Boston, MA.

51. Hawryluck L, Acharya SP, Shrestha GS. Critical care medicine in Nepal: before and after the massive earthquake and its aftershocks. World Federation of Societies of Intensive and Critical Care Medicine. Available at: http://www.world-critical-care.org/images/Critical_Care_Medicine_in_Nepal_World_federation_june_1st.pdf. Accessed August 6, 2020.

52. Giri S, Risnes K, Uleberg O, et al. Impact of 2015 earthquakes on a local hospital in Nepal: A prospective hospital-based study. PloS one 2018;13(2):e0192076.

53. Lehavi A, Meroz Y, Maryanovsky M, et al. Role of regional anaesthesia in disaster medicine: field hospital experience after the 2015 Nepal Earthquake. Eur J Anaesthesiol 2016;33:312–3.
54. Amatya S, Pal I, Chatterjee R. Assessment of coordination mechanism in 2015 Nepal earthquake, Kathmandu district. 2017. Available at: https://www.researchgate.net/publication/317041566_Assessment_of_Coordination_Mechanism_in_2015_Nepal_Earthquake_Kathmandu_District.
55. Goyet S, Rayamajhi R, Gyawali BN, et al. Post-earthquake health-service support, Nepal. Bull World Health Organ 2018;96(4):286.
56. World Meteorological Organization. Severe Weather Information Centre. Available at: https://severeweather.wmo.int/tc/cnp/acronyms.html#GTC. Accessed September 29, 2020.
57. National Oceanic and Atmospheric Administration. What is the difference between a hurricane and a typhoon? In Ocean Facts. Available at: https://oceanservice.noaa.gov/facts/cyclone.html. Accessed September 29, 2020.
58. Eddie P, Paul T. Natural Hazards: Causes and Effects Lesson 5- Tropical Cyclones. Prehosp Disaster Med 1995;10(3):202–16.
59. Windy app. How typhoon forms. Available at: https://windy.app/blog/how-typhoons-form.html. Accessed September 29, 2020.
60. International Pacific Research Center. More Typhoons Over the South China Sea? IPRC Clim 2005;5(2):3–5.
61. Hong Kong Observatory. The Year's Weather 2017. Available at: https://www.hko.gov.hk/en/wxinfo/pastwx/2017/ywx2017.htm. Accessed September 30, 2020.
62. Arcadis the Netherlands. Arcadis sustainable cities index 2015: Hong Kong has the highest natural disasters risk in Asia. Available at: http://www.arcadis-us.com/press/Hong_Kong_has_the_highest_natural_disasters_risk_in_Asia.aspx. Accessed September 30, 2020.
63. Hong Kong Observatory. The New 3-Tier Typhoon Classification. Available at: https://www.hko.gov.hk/en/aviat/outreach/product/20th/TCclass.htm. Accessed September 28, 2020.
64. Perez E, Thompson P. Natural hazards: causes and effects lesson 5 Prehosp Disaster Med 1995;10(3):202–15.
65. Campbell S. The history of wind damage in Hong Kong. APEC 21st Century COE short term Fellowship. Atsugi (Japan): Tokyo Polytechnic University; 2005.
66. World Health Organization. How hot weather affects health. Available at: https://www.euro.who.int/en/health-topics/environment-and-health/Climate-change/news/news/2013/7/how-hot-weather-affects-health. Accessed September 30, 2020.
67. Hong Kong Observatory. Super Typhoon Mangkhut. 1822. Available at: https://www.hko.gov.hk/en/informtc/mangkhut18/report.htm. Accessed September 28, 2020.
68. Hong Kong Legislative Council Secretariat. Council Business Division 2. Panel on Food Safety and Environmental Hygiene. Information note prepared by the Legislative Council Secretariat for the meeting on 13 November 2018. Post-typhoon follow-up efforts under the purview of the Food and Environmental Hygiene Department. Hong Kong Legislative Council Paper 7 November 2018 No. CB(2)207/18-19(06).
69. Kimmy Chung. How small Hong Kong hospital's emergency transfers defied might of Typhoon Mangkhut. South China Morning Post- Hong Kong- Health and Environment 22 September 2018.
70. Beigi R, Davis G, Hodges J, et al. Preparedness planning for pandemic influenza among large US maternity hospitals. Emerg Health Threats J 2009;2:e2.

71. JLL Singapore. How to prepare for a Super Typhoon. Available at: https://www.jll.com.sg/en/trends-and-insights/investor/how-to-prepare-for-a-super-typhoon. Accessed September 29, 2020.

72. Hong Kong Labour Department. Code of Practice in times of typhoons and rainstorms. 2020 April.

73. François-Xavier Bagnoud Center for Health and Human Rights Harvard T. H. Chan School of Public Health. Harvard University. Disaster Preparedness in Hong Kong. A Scoping Study. November 2016 (update).

74. Hick J, Einav S, Hanfling D, et al. Surge Capacity Principles. Care of the Critically Ill and Injured During Pandemics and Disasters: CHEST Consensus Statement. Chest 2014;146(4_Suppl):e1S–16S.

75. Soremekun OA, Zane RD, Walls A, et al. Cancellation of scheduled procedures as a mechanism to generate hospital bed surge capacity-a pilot study. Prehosp Disaster Med 2011;26(3):224–9.

76. Meites E, Farias D, Raffo L, et al. Hospital capacity during an influenza pandemic-Buenos Aires, Argentina, 2009. Infect Control Hosp Epidemiol 2011;32(1):87–90.

77. Horn RB, Kirsch TD. Disaster response 2.0: noncommunicable disease essential needs still unmet. Am J Public Health 2018;108(S3):S202–3.

78. Government of Hong Kong Special Administrative Region. Press Release. LCQ 20: Handling of fallen trees and broken branches. Available at: https://www.info.gov.hk/gia/general/201811/14/P2018111400452.htm. Accessed September 29, 2020.

Mass Casualty and the Role of the Anesthesiologist

Derek Nicholas Lodico, DO[a,b,*], Rear Admiral Darin Via, MD[b,c]

KEYWORDS

- Anesthesiologist • Austere medicine • Mass casualty incident
- Emergency preparedness • Mass disasters • Anesthesiologist role in conflict
- Resuscitation • Anesthesiologist triage

KEY POINTS

- Natural and man-made massive casualty events have been a part of our history, and injury patterns resembling those encountered on the battlefield are occurring with increased frequency.
- Understanding of how our modern emergency management systems have developed over time will help the anesthesiologist understand how their involvement is critical to the success of these programs.
- Global disasters and military armed conflict are different when it comes to the anesthesiologist's ethical decision-making process but provide a lesson-learned asset.
- Anesthesiologists are fundamental to the emergency management system, and their skills and daily routine make them key candidates as leaders and participants in the setting of a mass casualty incident.
- Anesthesiologists should feel a sense of obligation to self-educate, become members of their respective emergency management teams, and seek opportunities to develop and be involved with massive casualty training.

INTRODUCTION

Massive casualty events, whether on a small or large scale, have been reported throughout history. In most cases, they occur without warning. Many of the advances in the management of casualty care, especially on a scale that burdens a system, have come from past armed conflicts where the need for this care was anticipated. Key aspects of emergency preparedness, mitigation, planning, response, and recovery, are consistent with the primary role of the anesthesiologist.

[a] Naval Trauma Training Center, Los Angeles County + University of Southern California Medical Center, Keck School of Medicine, 1200 North State Street, Room 1050, Los Angeles, CA 90033, USA; [b] Uniformed Services University of Health Sciences, Bethesda, MD, USA; [c] Naval Medical Forces Atlantic, Navy Medicine East, 620 John Paul Jones Circle, Building 3, Suite 1400, Portsmouth, VA 23708, USA
* Corresponding author.
E-mail address: derek.n.lodico.mil@mail.mil

Anesthesiology Clin 39 (2021) 309–319
https://doi.org/10.1016/j.anclin.2021.03.001
1932-2275/21/Published by Elsevier Inc.
anesthesiology.theclinics.com

In developing and modern countries' medical systems, the anesthesiologist has varying roles in their integration and involvement with emergency management plans. The differences in these roles can be seen geographically, between smaller community-based hospitals and larger level I/II trauma centers, or simply based on dogma innate to the hospital's organization.[1–3] An anesthesiologist's training pathway and daily responsibility involve many of the key skill sets innate to all mass casualty management strategies. Management of personnel, awareness of available resources, ongoing triage, expertise in critical care management, and resuscitation are just a few of the skills expected of the anesthesiologist and represent essential elements of a modern emergency management system. Anesthesiologists should be involved with all aspects of emergency preparedness and take an active role to self-educate, be involved with, and develop programs within their institution. In lieu of more recent mass casualty events, the arguments that "this will not happen where I live" or "I don't work in a trauma hospital" are not valid arguments to avoid active involvement in emergency preparedness plans, including mass casualty event management strategies.

DEFINITION

The World Health Organization (WHO) defines a disaster as "[a] sudden event causing severe destruction of infrastructure, people and the economy and which overwhelms the resources of that country, region, or community."[4] The Inter-Agency Contingency Planning Guidelines for Humanitarian Assistance defines emergency preparedness as "actions taken in anticipation of an emergency to facilitate rapid, effective and appropriate response to the situation."[4] A mass casualty incident is defined as "an event which generates more patients at one time than locally available resources can manage using routine procedures. It requires exceptional emergency arrangements and additional or extraordinary assistance."[5] This disaster could be as little as 5 patients, for a small military combat surgical team or community-based rural hospital, or as many as 50 to 100 patients for a level I trauma center.

The WHO has developed an Emergency Medical Team Classification and Program.[6] Within these guidelines, it defines the role of the anesthesiologist and delineates that any organization deploying a level 2 field hospital must provide at least 1 medically qualified anesthesiologist.[6] It also points out the differences between using a nurse anesthetist and an anesthesiologist. Both can provide anesthesia, but only the anesthesiologist has the expertise with regards to physician-based perioperative and critical care management.

As seen with the recent COVID-19 disaster and response, anesthesiologists were called on to act as critical care physicians.[7] Even without a formal intensive care training, general anesthesiologists are expected to be able to manage critically ill patients for a prolonged period of time. With the potential for damage to medical infrastructure as a result of a natural or man-made disaster, the anesthesiologist plays a pivotal role with regards to prolonged field care. Thus, an anesthesiologist may provide not only austere intraoperative care but also prolonged critical care until evacuation is possible. These WHO scenarios of "level 2" care parallel the current military doctrine with regards to Role 2 care.

Role 2 care is defined by US military doctrine as a scenario of limited hospital capability, consisting of advanced damage control resuscitation and surgery provided by a small, mobile, forward-positioned medical treatment facility and surgical team[8] (**Fig. 1**). Role 2 care challenges the anesthesiologist to overcome the austere environment lacking in resources with which they are accustomed.

HISTORY

Massive casualty events have been recorded throughout history and may be either natural or man-made. Indeed, the beginnings of many of the large-scale emergency management systems throughout the world can be linked to single large-scale events, such as earthquakes, floods, hurricanes, tornados, and fires.[9,10] In contrast to natural events that come with little or no warning, armed conflicts may be able to anticipate casualties that may overwhelm the resources and ability to provide treatment.

Triage, a word known well to all anesthesiologists, is an integral part of mass casualty management, and it has a detailed history. Derived from the French "to thin out," it has also been used by the Japanese and British referencing the sorting of beans and wools, respectively.[11] The origin of its use with respect to medicine dates back to the Napoleonic Wars of the early nineteenth century, credited to Drs Dominique Jean Larrey and Pierre Francois Percy.[12–15] Dr Larrey realized there was no organized method of dealing with battlefield injuries and went on with Dr Percy to develop a field ambulance and sorting system.

Physician involvement in mass casualty events dates to ancient Roman times. The Romans were one of the first groups reported to have physicians specifically assigned to the treatment of battle injuries.[16] Much of the progress in battlefield medicine was lost during the dark ages and resumed with more modern warfare in Europe, as discussed above. One of the first mentions of anesthesia for mass casualty situations was in the latter half of the nineteenth century. A Russian surgeon, Nikolai Ivanovich Pirogov, was one of the first to systematically provide modern medical care for mass casualty incidents. Dr Pirogov realized that battlefield injuries needed early and specialized care and is credited as the first to use chloroform anesthesia during surgery on the battlefield.[17,18]

Developments in modern disaster medicine were initially shaped in the 1950s around the potential for mass casualties from atomic war.[19] In the 1960s, Dr Joseph R. Schaeffer, a colonel and physician, contributed to the development of disaster medicine. A consultant on disaster medicine to the American Medical Association and the American College of Surgeons, Dr Schaeffer was directly involved in disaster management during Hurricane Carla in 1961, an event involving the management and care of 20,000 evacuated residents.[20] His experience revealed how little first aid education the general public received. As a result, Dr Schaeffer dedicated much of his time to disaster medicine planning.

THE ROLE OF THE ANESTHESIOLOGIST IN MASS CASUALTY AND TRAUMA

The anesthesiologist may view themselves as having only a perioperative role in the event of a mass casualty incident, but as human resources are consumed, providers will need to adapt to multiple roles. The emergency department of even the most robust level I/II trauma centers has its limit of beds and providers. Some of the triage

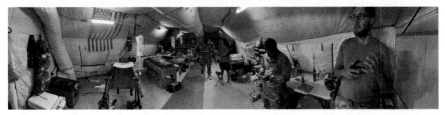

Fig. 1. Role 2 austere resuscitative surgical care unit, Syria. (Photo Dr. Derek Lodico CDR/MC/USN.)

may need to be done in hallways, lobbies, drop-off circles, or converted hospital wards.

The Egyptian revolution in January 2011, which started as a peaceful protest, ended in violent clashes with security forces, resulting in 846 deaths and 6400 injuries.[21] Cairo University Hospital, the oldest and largest hospital in Egypt, was in the heart of these protests. The hospital's 5500-bed capacity and 72 operating rooms (ORs) were crippled as a result of a telecommunications shut down by the government. Furthermore, the hospital was staffed with a skeleton crew before the violent events outside with only 8 ORs running. The hospital was quickly the center of a mass casualty incident when more than 3000 injured patients arrived. Of the admitted patients, 339 needed urgent surgical care within 6 hours of arrival. All security forces for the hospital were diverted to the ensuing conflict, and as such, were unavailable to the hospital.

The resuscitation bays were overrun with patients and family members. The decision was made to use the attending anesthesiologists and deploy them to the resuscitation rooms to triage and disposition patients to the surgical intensive care unit. At the time of this event, 8 anesthesiologists, 4 of which were residents, and 19 surgeons were on call. Ten volunteer anesthesiologists eventually arrived to assist, but the number of urgent surgical cases forced many of the anesthesiologists to staff 2 operations simultaneously with house officer assistance. There was no involvement of the anesthesiologist in the hospital's mass casualty plan before this event.

Today, anesthesiologists perform triage on a regular basis. In the preoperative clinic, patients are triaged in order to determine the need of further workup and appropriateness of the surgery based on their presenting state of health. Patients are triaged the day of surgery to determine if they are appropriate to go forward with surgery, and then a continual triage process takes place in real time during an operative case. Being on call, managing urgent and emergent cases, assessing critical airway and respiratory emergencies, and managing the operative room board in a busy hospital require continuous assessment and can be compared with the triage necessary during a mass casualty incident.

Flexibility is one of the anesthesiologist's most important qualities. Very often a plan for anesthesia is altered or disrupted by patient and/or surgical factors requiring real-time adjustments. Often procedures are conducted outside of the main OR in remote spaces, necessitating the adaptability of the anesthesiologist. Unanticipated equipment failure may occur during the course of an intraoperative case requiring quick recognition and correction, both cornerstone qualities. Mass casualty incidents will never occur on our terms and may necessitate using fieldlike settings in the event that our medical infrastructure is damaged or crippled.

After the 2010 earthquake in Haiti, an already underdeveloped medical care infrastructure was almost completely disabled. Medical relief came in the form of Role 2 field hospitals[22,23] (**Fig. 2**). In the US military setting, a Role 2 light footprint field surgical unit has become the new norm with regards to combat trauma medicine. A review of the surgical care provided during the wars in Iraq and Afghanistan from 2001 to 2012 concluded that early use of a tourniquet, immediate availability of blood, and quick transport to surgical care resulted in reduction in mortality by 44%.[24–26] In order to have surgical care available, these surgical units need to be in proximity to the point of injury. These teams need to be mobile, to have the ability to set up expeditiously, and to carry the operative resources with them to perform damage control resuscitation and surgery.

All branches of the US armed forces have a form of a Role 2 surgical team.[27] The military service doctrine that dictates their role and capabilities varies. The teams

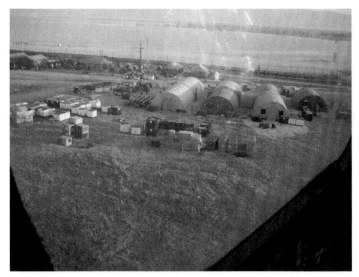

Fig. 2. Field hospital for Haiti Earthquake Disaster Relief 2010. (Photo taken by Dr. Adam Cooper, CDR/MC/USN.)

that have the lightest footprint have the biggest challenge, and the anesthesiologist will have their flexibility and willingness to adapt put to the greatest test in these scenarios. The challenges that the anesthesiologist faces as part of a US military Role 2 surgical team are similar to what may be seen in a Role 2 field hospital setting on the civilian side. As an example, the US Navy has a Role 2 light maneuver combat surgical team (R2LM). The R2LM is traditionally composed of an anesthesiologist or certified registered nurse anesthetist, a surgeon, an emergency room (ER) physician, a respiratory therapist, an intensive care unit nurse, an ER nurse, 1 to 2 surgical technicians, and a medic (hospital corpsman). The composition of this team may be adjusted based on available manpower and objective. The current doctrine describes that the team has the ability to provide damage control resuscitation for 4 patients with the ability to perform damage control surgery on 2 of the 4 patients and on-going care for up to 18 to 96 hours. The capability to take care of additional patients and provide prolonged field care will vary based on resources and supplies. This doctrine and team composition may vary depending on the scenario and the environment.

All the surgical and resuscitative gear can be packed into 9 roller bags that can be worn as a backpack in its most scalable form (**Fig. 3**). The weight of each bag is approximately 60 pounds. Power is provided by a solar rechargeable battery pack or small gas-powered generators. All the equipment used is lightweight and tactical. Ventilation is accomplished using a Zole 731 (Zole Medical Corporation, Chelmsford, MA, USA) tactical ventilator, which operates on battery power for up to 10 hours. This ventilator has all of the traditional settings of an intensive care unit ventilator and can be used for surgery and follow up care. Its rugged design can tolerate a depth of 609.6 meters below sea level and elevation up to 7620 meters; it is approved for en route care via helicopter or other transportation platform. Traditional oxygen sources with a minimum of 55 psi are compatible, as is oxygen from a cylinder. In the field, oxygen concentrators are used and can provide up to 3 L per minute of flow. Using a Douglass reservoir bag in this case can produce a continuous inhaled oxygen concentration in the 60% range.

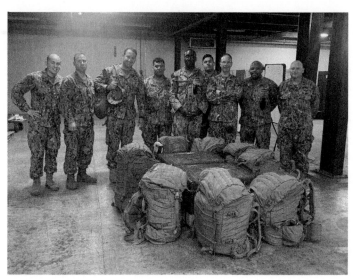

Fig. 3. Expiditionary Resuscitative Surgical Care Team 22 Light Packout. (Photo taken by Dr. Derek Lodico, CDR/MC/USN.)

The availability of blood and surgical capability define a Role 2. Blood is available to the R2LM in multiple locations around the world and is transported via temperature-controlled devices. A blood transport container (Combat Medical, Harrisburg, NC, USA) has been developed that allows for the maintenance of whole blood, packed red cells, or plasma, at or less than 8°C for up to 120 hours. These tactical, smaller, insulated containers can carry up to 6 units of whole blood, and up to 4 of these containers can be carried with the roller bags described earlier. Blood warming is accomplished using the Warrior Extreme (QinFlow, Plano, TX, USA), which will deliver 4 to 5 units of blood on 1 battery charge and heats up to 38°C in 11 seconds. Although not a traditional method of blood product warming, a SousVide (Eades Appliance Technology LLC, Broomfield, CO, USA) (**Fig. 4**) device can be used in the field to heat additional units of blood following AABB guidelines.[28]

Arterial and venous blood gas samples can be measured using an I-STAT point-of-care device (Abbott Point of Care Inc, Princeton, NJ, USA) using one of the multiple laboratory panel cartridges (ie, CG8$^+$). A small portable ultrasound is available for point-of-care ultrasound. End-tidal CO_2 continuous monitoring is accomplished using the EMMA Portable Real-Time Capnography (Masimo Corporation, Irvine, CA, USA), which is small and pocket portable and attaches directly to the endotracheal tube. Dial-a-flow infusion tubing is used to titrate intravenous (IV) medications to effect. Although this gravity-fed method for IV solutions is older and has been replaced with safer infusion pumps, this dial-a-flow method has been revisited in the COVID-19 era with the shortages of infusion pump devices. The Institute for Safe Medical Practices published a review article regarding the planning for anticipated shortages of smart pumps to include the use of dial-a-flow IV infusion tubing as an alternative.[29]

There is not a volatile gas component/delivery system taken with these smaller units, although there are options available to the US military for smaller volatile anesthesia delivery systems.[30] The anesthesia provided for surgery is via regional anesthesia and total intravenous anesthesia. Medications used for surgery rely heavily on ketamine as the primary anesthetic and vecuronium as the paralytic. During the 2013

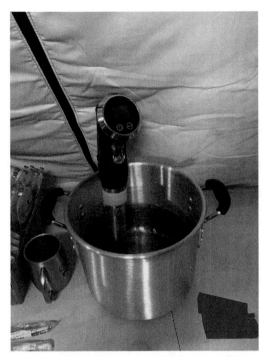

Fig. 4. A SousVide used as a blood warming bath during austere field conditions. (Photo taken by Dr. Derek Lodico, CDR/MC/USN.)

response to the earthquake in Haiti, 90% of all general anesthetics were performed using ketamine versus 10% under inhalation anesthetic.[31] Ketamine can be transported without refrigeration, has the desired properties of anesthesia and analgesia, and comes in concentrated vials. Ketamine is a rugged, effective, and portable anesthetic agent. Other benefits include maintenance of respiratory drive and minimal cardiovascular depression. Ketamine can be incorporated into a drip for postoperative pain management and sedation. Vecuronium comes in a vial in powder form, allowing for transport without refrigeration. Propofol is included in the formulary but seldom used secondary to its temperature lability, bulk, and negative hemodynamic effects. Although it could prove useful for postoperative sedation in a hemodynamically stable patient, a mixture of an opiate, ketamine, and paralytic may be the best option until evacuation. The usefulness of regional anesthesia has been demonstrated during disaster responses and is also used, is effective, and has been found to be the desired method by providers for postoperative pain control in the austere environment.[22,32,33]

Team leadership and communication in a mass casualty incident have been sighted as being as important as medical knowledge and cognitive ability.[34] Anesthesiologists are accustomed to directing a team in the care of operative patients in the perioperative period. In France, anesthesiologists play an important leadership role not only in the OR but also in the prehospital and emergency preparedness response team. For 30+ years, anesthesiologists have been part of France's emergency medical service called Service d'Aide Medicale Urgente (SAMU). On November 13, 2015, multiple terrorist attacks were carried out in Paris at the same time. SAMU was mobilized to areas where fire and rescue first responders were at the point of injury. Upon arrival on scene, anesthesiologists were involved with the triage and on-site patient management. In addition, at the area hospitals receiving these patients, anesthesiologists were a part of the receiving teams located outside of the OR. Pitie-Salpetriere Hospital treated 302 patients during the hours following these attacks. Upon arrival, patients were met by a team consisting of an anesthesiologist, surgeon, fellows, and nurses that directed patients either to the emergency department or to trauma units based on presentation.[35]

CHALLENGES

Despite all good intent by the individual provider and hospital systems as a whole, there are still many gaps in the system when it comes to mass casualty and disaster management. The WHO cites that one of the largest gaps is that many countries have not developed mass casualty management plans.[4] The WHO emphasizes the need to address this issue at all levels starting with the individual. Just having knowledge that your hospital has a mass casualty management plan will enhance the ability of the individual to respond appropriately in the event that it is activated, while minimizing stress and anxiety.

The anesthesiologist is frequently alone on call in a community-based hospital. In this scenario, there is a false sense of confidence that a few phone calls to other medical providers can manage any surgical or resuscitative problem. With proper planning and a mass casualty management plan in place, this can be true. In the mass shooting incident in Las Vegas on October 1, 2017, one of the primary hospitals where the shooting victims arrived was not a level I/II trauma center. The skeleton staff on call was quickly overwhelmed with patients. They did have an emergency response plan and ultimately a total of 215 penetrating gunshot wounds were seen, and within 6 hours, they did 28 damage-control surgeries and 67 surgeries total within the first 24 hours. Staff were quoted as saying that the knowledge of the plan's existence was beneficial.[36]

In 2005, a survey was conducted to include 135 accredited US anesthesiology residency programs. Ninety percent of the programs responded, and of those, only 37% of the responders stated that they had any type of training to handle patients inflicted with weapons of mass destruction.[37] In 2013, an online survey was conducted to include the anesthesia attendings and residents from the Johns Hopkins Hospital in Baltimore, Maryland, the University of Oklahoma Health Sciences Center in Oklahoma City, Oklahoma, and the University of Washington Medical Center in Seattle, Washington. The questions were formulated to assess the perspectives regarding disaster medicine and public health preparedness. The results concluded that a minority of the attending and few residents thought that their program provided them with adequate disaster preparation and training. Greater than 85% of the attendings and 70% of the residents thought that their programs should provide them with preparation and training with regards to disaster medicine.[38]

Disasters and events resulting in mass casualty incidents will continue to play a role in the life of the anesthesiologist. By nature of their training, anesthesiologists are specialists in trauma medicine. Although there are no Accreditation Council for Graduate Medical Education (ACGME)-approved anesthesiology trauma fellowships, there are several programs in the United States that offer trauma training outside of a residency in anesthesiology. In addition, some anesthesiology residency programs are stronger than others when it comes to exposing their residents to trauma and burn medicine. With no ACGME-specific requirement for exposure of residents to trauma and burns, the responsibility falls on us to ensure that we receive the necessary training and exposure. In addition, it is our responsibility to ensure that we maintain our own "readiness," so in the event of an unforeseen disaster, we are ready to respond.

This is not the first publication to bring attention to the value the anesthesiologist brings to the emergency management team and disaster preparedness.[28] Although there are geographic differences when it comes to the extent of involvement or role the anesthesiologist plays within their institution's emergency preparedness teams, we must start by being proactive. As anesthesiologists, we must ask about our own institution's plans in the event of a disaster. In the event the number of injured patients overwhelm our capabilities, we must ask what we can do to help. Programs such as "Stop the Bleed," Advanced Trauma Life Support, prehospital trauma life support, and disaster management and emergency preparedness training are all significant and will lead to improvements in your personal and institution's preparedness for unforeseen future challenges.

DISCLAIMER

"The views expressed in this article reflect the results of research conducted by the author and do not necessarily reflect the official policy or position of the Department of the Navy, Department of Defense, nor the United States Government."

CLINICS CARE POINTS

- Response Objectives and basic strategies are the same for every incident; however the approach will vary depending on available resources and the situation.
- Patient distribution to the appropriate healthcare facility is a component of triage and will effect survival.

DISCLOSURE

The authors have nothing to disclose.

REFERENCES

1. Kristiasnsen T, Soreide K, Ringdal KG, et al. Trauma systems and early management of severe injuries in Scandinavia: review of the current state. Injury 2010;42: 444–52.
2. Carlli PA, Riou B, Barriot P. Trauma anesthesia practices throughout the world: France. In: Texbook of trauma anesthesia and critical care. St Louis, MO: Mosby-Year Book Inc; 1993. p. 199–204 [Chapter 17].
3. Rognas L, Hansen TM, Kirkland H, et al. Pre-hospital advanced airway management by experienced anesthesiologists: a prospective descriptive study. Scand J Trauma Rescu Emerg Med 2013;21:58.
4. WHO. Humanitarian health action. Glossary of humanitarian terms. Available at: http://www.who.int/hac/about/definitions/en/. Accessed 01 October 2020.
5. WHO. Mass casualty management systems. Available at: https://www.who.int/hac/techguidance/MCM_inside_Jul07.pdf. Accessed October 01, 2020.
6. Norton I, von Schreeb J, Aitken P, et al. WHO. Classification and minimum standards for foreign medical teams in sudden onset disasters 2013. Available at: www.who.int/hac/global_health_cluster/fmt_guidelines_september2013.pdf. Accessed October 01, 2020.

7. Cheney C. Analysis-coronavirus: how to redeploy anesthesiology resources to the ICU setting. Available at: https://www.healthleadersmedia.com/clinical-care/coronavirus-how-redeploy-anesthesiology-resources-icu-setting.   Accessed October 03, 2020.

8. Kotwal RS, Staudt AM, Trevino JD, et al. A review of casualties transported to Role 2 medical treatment facilities in Afghanistan. Mil Med 2018;183(suppl_1):134–45.

9. Cracow Emergency Medical Services. Homepage. Available at: http://www.kpr.med.pl. Accessed October 03, 2020.

10. Page J. A brief history of EMS. JEMS 1989;14:S11.

11. Nakao H, Ukai I, Kotani J. A review of the history of the origin of triage from a disaster medicine perspective. Acute Med Surg 2017;4(4):379–84.

12. Baker R, Strosberg M. Triage and equality: an historical reassessment of utilitarian analyses of triage. Kennedy Inst Ethics J 1992;2(2):103–23.

13. Balgg RC. Triage: Napoleon to the present day. J Nephrol 2004;17:629–32.

14. Robbertson-Steel I. Evolution of triage systems. Emerg Med J 2006;23:154–5.

15. Remba SJ, Varon J, Rivera A, et al. Dominique Jean Larrey (1766-1842). Med Pregfl 2011;64:97–100.

16. Peters S. The hospitalized legionnaire at the Rhine front at the outset of the Roman Principate. Wurzbg Medizinhist Mitt 2010;29:158–93.

17. Ring A. Nikolaj Pirogov: a pioneer of modern surgery. Chirurg 2011;82:164–8.

18. Sorokina T. The great Russian surgeon Nikolay Ivanovich Pirogov (1810-1881). Versalius 2011;17:10–5.

19. United Press. Hard role for doctor seen in atomic war. Reno Evening Gaz 1955;30.

20. Williams J. Disaster medicine: a history. Am J Disaster Med 2008;03:124–30.

21. Mukhtar A, Hasanin A, El-Adawy A, et al. The friday of rage of the egyptian revolution: a unique role for anesthesiologists. Anesthesia and Analgesia 2012;114(4):862–5.

22. Morey TE, Rice MJ. Anesthesia in an austere setting-lessons learned from the Haiti relief operation. Anesthesiol Clin 2013;31:107–15.

23. Ginzburg E, O'Neill W, Goldschmidt-Clermont P, et al. Rapid medical relief-Project Medishare and the Haitian earthquake. N Engl J Med 2010;362:e31.

24. Howard JT, Kotwal RS, Stern CA, et al. Use of combat casualty care data to assess the US military trauma system during the Afghanistan and Iraq conflicts, 2001-2017. JAMA Surg 2019;154(7):600–8.

25. Lane I, Stockinger Z, Sauer S, et al. The Afghan theater: a review of military medical doctrine from 2008 to 2014. Mil Med 2017;182(S1):32–40.

26. Stockinger ZT, Holcomb JB, Nessen SC, et al. A US military Role 2 forward surgical team database study of combat mortality in Afghanistan. J Trauma Acute Care Surg 2018;85(3):603–12.

27. Gross MJ. Office of the Air Force Surgeon General fellowship paper –damage control surgery and the joint solution. Submitted to HQ AF/SG35X, Defense Headquarters, Falls Church, VA. Available at: https://apps/dtic.mil/dtic/tr/fulltext/u2/1042216.pdf. Accessed October 10, 2020.

28. Kuza C, McIsaac J. Role of the anesthesiologist during mass casualty events. Am Soc Anesth Monit 2017;81(4):14–7.

29. O'Connell S. Planning for anticipated shortages of smart infusion pumps and dedicated administration sets. Institute for Safe Medication Practices; 2020. Available at: https://ismp.org/resources/planning-anticipated-shortage-smart-infusion-pumps-and-dedicated-administration-sets. Accessed October 12, 2020.

30. No authors listed. Anesthesia systems for ambulatory surgery settings. Health Devices 2006 Aug;35(8):316–29.

31. Rice M, Gwertzman A, Finley T, et al. Anaesthetic practice in Haiti after the 2010 earthquake. Anesth Analg 2010;111:1445–9.

32. Mathais Q, Montcriol A, Cotte J, et al. Anesthesia during deployment of a military forward surgical unit in low income countries: a register study of 1547 anesthesia cases. PLoS One 2019;14(10):e0223497.

33. Buckenmaier CC 3rd, Lee EH, Shields CH, et al. Regional anesthesia in austere environments. Reg Anesth Pain Med 2003;28:321–7.

34. King RV, Larkin GL, Fowler RL, et al. Characteristics of effective disaster responders and leaders: a survey of disaster medical practitioners. Disaster Med Public Health Prep 2016;10(5):720–3.

35. Hirsch M, Carli P, Nizard R, et al. The medical response to multisite terrorist attacks in Paris. The Lancet 2015;386:2535–8.

36. Kuhls DA, Fildes JJ, Johnson M, et al. Southern Nevada Trauma System uses proven techniques to save lives after 1 October shooting. Chicago (IL): American College of Surgeons Bulletin; 2018. Available at: https://bulletin.facs.org/2018/03/southern-nevada-trauma-system-uses-proven-techniques-to-save-lives-after-1-october-shooting/. Accessed on October 15, 2020.

37. King RV, Larkin GL, Fowler RL, et al. Characteristics of effective disaster responders and leaders: a survey of disaster medical practitioners. Disaster Med Public Health Prep 2016;10(5):720–3.

38. Hayanga HK, Barnett DJ, Shallow NR, et al. Anesthesiologists and disaster medicine: a needs assessment for education and training and reported willingness to respond. Anesth Analg 2017;124(5):1662–9.

Battlefield Medicine
Anesthesia and Critical Care in the Combat Zone

J. Michael Jaeger, PhD, MD[a],*, Darian C. Rice, MD, PhD[b,1],
Brooke Albright-Trainer, MD[b,c]

KEYWORDS

- Combat casualty care • TCCC • Joint Trauma System • Battlefield anesthesia
- Aeromedical evacuation

KEY POINTS

- Combat medicine requires all physicians regardless of primary specialty to be capable of managing a spectrum of injuries and diseases under austere and hostile conditions.
- The Joint Trauma System is a hierarchy of combat casualty care that mitigates the limited resources and harsh conditions of the battlefield to ensure the best possible care for combatants.
- Anesthesiologists play a vital role in this system at multiple levels, managing large numbers of injuries as well as unfamiliar diseases.
- Multimodality pain management is an important aspect of their practice.
- The Critical Care Aeromedical Transport team has become an essential link in the chain of survival from the theater of operations through to continental United States.

The practice of medicine in a foreign, austere, combat setting requires a great deal from its practitioners. Although the patient population is generally young and healthy, war generates horrific injuries, frequently in large numbers over short intervals. When coupled with unfamiliar diseases that can appear whenever public health infrastructure is destroyed or never existed, every member of the medical team must exercise a wider range of medical skills and knowledge. In addition, everyone must be creative, adaptable, and demonstrate resilience to perform continuously under duress, something not typically experienced during peacetime at home. Our goal is to describe the manner in which our current military medical system operates in a combat environment with a particular emphasis on what the anesthesiologist and intensivist should expect to experience.

[a] Departments of Anesthesiology and Surgery, Division of Critical Care Medicine, University of Virginia Health System, Box 800710, Charlottesville, VA 22908, USA; [b] Department of Anesthesiology, Division of Critical Care Medicine, University of Virginia Health System, Box 800710, Charlottesville, VA 22908, USA; [c] Department of Anesthesiology, Central Virginia VA HCS, Richmond, VA 23249, USA
[1] He is also a Navy Reservist currently serving with Naval Medical Center Portsmouth, VA.
* Corresponding author.
E-mail address: jmj4w@virginia.edu

Anesthesiology Clin 39 (2021) 321–336
https://doi.org/10.1016/j.anclin.2021.03.002
1932-2275/21/© 2021 Elsevier Inc. All rights reserved.

anesthesiology.theclinics.com

THE MODERN US MILITARY JOINT TRAUMA SYSTEM
Progress in Combat Casualty Care

Progress in combat casualty care is the direct result of improvements in the management of casualties from the point of wounding through reconstructive surgery and rehabilitation. A hierarchy of care has been developed within component services of the US military, called the Joint Trauma System, which enables progressively sophisticated levels of care and a process for patient transport thorough the system anywhere in the world.

The success of this approach can be seen in the improvement in combat casualty statistics over the past 100 years (**Table 1**). Definition of casualty statistics:

- WIA (wounded in action) – is the total number of injured on the battlefield that are unable to temporarily or permanently return to duty.
- KIA (killed in action) – is the number of combat *deaths that occur before* reaching a medical treatment facility (MTF).
- DOW (died of wounds) – is the number of combat injured that *died after reaching* an MTF.

To understand the impact of interventions in combat medicine and combatant protection, Holcomb, and colleagues,[1] stated that it is imperative to define "case fatality rates," which is the fraction of an exposed group (all those wounded in action including all those who die (anywhere along the continuum) expressed as a percent. In their analysis of fatalities on the battlefield from 2001 to 2011, Eastridge and colleagues[2] determined that, for those KIA, 35% of the deaths were deemed instantaneous and another 52% occurred within minutes to hours before arrival at an MTF. For casualties making it to an MTF, 12.7% died of wounds overall. The general distribution of injury mechanisms was 14% (explosives), 22% (gunshot wounds), and 4.2% (a mix of motor vehicle accidents, crush injuries, or industrial accidents). Enemy tactics and the increasing lethality of weapons have certainly changed the nature of injury and the degree of devastation. Countering this reality are the improvements in body armor, adaptive countertactics, mine-resistant armored vehicles, field care, casualty evacuation, and capability of far-forward MTFs. Therefore, the anesthesiologist might expect greater numbers surviving to the MTF, that is, a potential decrease in KIA for those with potentially survivable injuries, but more grievously injured presenting to MTFs with higher likelihood of died of wounds. When corrected for case fatality rates, the data indicate an overall gain in survival for our combat casualties today. As of December 2017, the published data for Afghanistan and Iraq define an overall case fatality rates of 8.6% and 10.1%, respectively.[3] Of note, a recent separate analysis of 29,958 casualties from Afghanistan and Iraq from 2003 through 2014 found nonbattle injuries responsible for 34.1% of the total casualties and 11.5% of all deaths.[4] The leading mechanisms of nonbattle injuries were falls (21.3%), motor vehicle accidents (18.8%), industrial-type accidents (12.6%), blunt objects (10.8%), self-inflicted gunshot wounds (7.1%), and sports (6.8%), which serves to emphasize the complexity of the problem and, more important, the difficulty in implementing troop protection in combat zones.

THE NATURE OF COMBAT WOUNDS IN CURRENT CONFLICTS

Anesthesiologists and intensivists need to be familiar with the types of injuries that combatants encounter and prepare accordingly. Given the current enemy tactics, injuries from high explosives, for example, improvised explosive devices, either person borne or vehicle borne, have been described as a signature injury of the past 20 years.

Table 1
A comparison of US Mortality data for medical treatment facilities (1898 to October 2005)

	Spanish-American War	World War I	World War II	Korean War	Vietnam War	Iraq and Afghanistan (OIF/OEF) October 2001 to October 2005
KIA	2446 [total deaths (not delineated)]	11,516 [total deaths (not delineated)]	152,359 (ground troops only)	36,568 [total deaths (not delineated)]	38,281 (ground troops only)	1266 (ground troops only)
DOW	—	—	20,810 (ground troops only)	—	4983 (ground troops only)	383 (ground troops only)
WIA	—	—	752,396 (ground troops only)	—	235,398 (ground troops only)	16,235 (ground troops only)
Total number serving	306,760	4,734,991	16,112,566	5,720,000	8,744,000	—
% KIA	—	—	20.2	—	20.0	13.8
% DOW	—	—	3.5	—	3.2	4.8
CFR	—	—	19.1	—	15.8	9.4

Abbreviations: CFR, case fatality rate; DOW, died of wounds; KIA, killed in action; WIA, wounded in action.
Data are compiled from and Tables 1 and 3 in ref.[1] and Table 1 in ref.[34] Note that the data in % rows is for *ground combat troops only* from Table 3, ref.[1]
Data from Holcomb JB, Stansbury LG, Champion HR, et al. Understanding combat casualty care statistics. J Trauma 2006;60:397-401 and Pruitt, Jr BA. Combat casualty and surgical progress. Ann Surg 2006;243(6):715-29.

However, rocket-propelled grenades, landmines, rockets, and mortars are also prevalent, depending on the combat theater. Most deaths on the battlefield are caused by total body disruption, severe brain injury, or severe hemorrhage, and have little chance of survival. However, the severity of these injuries are a continuum and the lesser injured individuals can survive to reach an MTF and in large numbers. An improvised explosive device casualty can suffer from several different types of penetrating and blast-related blunt or thermal injuries that usually involve multiple body regions. One analysis of all types of combat injuries calculated an average of 4.2 wounds per casualty.[5] Partial dismemberment clearly results in significant blood loss and requires prompt resuscitation. Additional injuries often associated with the pelvic and extremity avulsions are traumatic brain injuries, ocular injuries, burns, and abdominal (visceral disruption or vascular) or chest (visceral contusion/laceration or vascular) wounds. Maxillofacial injuries may present a potentially compromised and challenging airway.[6,7] Because the primary blast over pressure wave can transmit rapid pressure changes through airspaces in the human body, any air-filled bowel, lungs, middle ear, and sinuses can be at risk for rupture. Rapid assessment and reassessment while treating the identified problems is essential because these injuries can evolve. Careful selection of adjunct drug therapy and anesthetics in the face of shock and a complex injury pattern is paramount. A focused ultrasound examination can be helpful to assess rapidly for pneumothorax or hemothorax, cardiac injury, volume state, and intra-abdominal hemorrhage.

Gunshot wounds from military full metal-jacketed bullets produce varying degrees of tissue damage depending on their muzzle velocity, distance of flight, any deflection upon striking their target, and organs penetrated. The high muzzle velocities of most military arms ensure a greater stable trajectory over longer distances with a greater chance of penetration.[8] Passage of the bullet through soft tissue creates a temporary cavity that crushes and shears tissue, but also leaves behind a relative negative pressure zone that can suck bacteria and foreign material into the wound. Denser tissues like the liver, kidney, muscle, or heart suffer far more extensive damage from cavitation than elastic, less dense tissues like the lung. The degree of tissue damage also depends on the induction of tumbling or fragmentation of the round when it enters body tissues and transfers kinetic energy. Finally, deflection of the bullet, for example, after striking bone, can cause the bullet to veer in any direction and enter adjacent body cavities.[8,9]

Shock, acidosis, and hypothermia are a byproduct of hemorrhage and tissue destruction that contributes to the trauma-induced coagulopathy that is frequently associated with severe combat wounds.[10–13] Early and thoughtful resuscitation following accepted damage-control resuscitation guidelines is recommended.[13,14] The 4 basic components of damage-control resuscitation are:

- Hypotensive resuscitation (pre-MTF), whereby normalization of blood pressure is delayed until control of hemorrhage is ensured.
- Damage control surgery, where the focus is abbreviated surgery to rapidly obtain control of hemorrhage and contamination with definitive surgery delayed until a stable physiology has been restored.
- Limited use of intravenous crystalloids and colloids, which may worsen coagulopathy through dilution of clotting factors and have proinflammatory effects.
- A balanced approach to blood product transfusion; fresh whole blood is preferable, but transfusion of packed red cells, fresh frozen plasma, and platelets in a 1:1:1 ratio improves outcomes and reverses the acute coagulopathy of trauma.[13–18]

These principles may require slight modification in a combat setting in that geography, weather, enemy activity, and long casualty evacuation distances may force some adjustments in the pre-MTF phase.[18]

ROLE I OF THE JOINT TRAUMA SYSTEM: "BATTLEFIELD CASUALTY CARE"

The first phase of the response to the injured combatant at the point of wounding involves self-aid, buddy-aid, Combat Lifesaver (designated nonmedical combatant with enhanced first aid training), and treatment by designated Army Medics (91W), Navy Corpsmen, USAF Independent Duty Medical Technician, or Pararescuemen (PJ). The degree of medical training and experience can vary greatly, from basic combatant field first aid to basic Navy corpsmen or Army combat medic (91W; 6 weeks, basic emergency medical technician). Most special operations medics, corpsmen, and PJs, for example, Special Forces Medical Sergeant (18D), undergo over 12 months of specialized training and are the equivalent of National Registry of Emergency Medical Technicians–paramedic. These individuals have the difficult task of providing the initial assessment, treatment, and triage while under hostile fire in any terrain (including urban) and in any weather.

When feasible, evacuation can proceed from the battlefield to either an Army Battalion Aid Station (BAS) or Marine Shock Trauma Platoon. At this level, care is provided by a physician assistant and/or general medical officer or emergency medical physician capable of providing initial resuscitation and advanced trauma life support as well as basic sick call.[19]

TACTICAL COMBAT CASUALTY CARE

In 1989, a Naval Special Warfare Biomedical Research Program was initiated with a broad agenda which included improving combat casualty care for US Navy SEALs in the field.[20] The project was spearheaded by Captain Frank K. Butler, Jr, MC, USN (a former Vietnam SEAL/UDT) and quickly expanded to include senior medical officers and enlisted medical personnel representing the US Special Operations Command units and the Uniformed Services University of the Health Sciences. Their efforts were published as the Tactical Combat Casualty Care (TCCC) Guidelines in 1996.[21] Its purpose was to reduce casualties and minimize morbidity yet still accomplish the tactical mission. TCCC was initially aimed at US Special Operations Command, that is, the SEAL corpsman, Special Forces medical sergeant (18D), Ranger Combat Medic, and Air Force PJ, providing the primary aid to an injured comrade while actively engaged in hostile action frequently in very remote, austere conditions with limited support from conventional forces. It divided the process into 3 phases: (1) care under fire, (2) tactical field care, and (3) tactical evacuation (TACEVAC), with each phase as defined in **Table 2**.[21] Documented success of the program over the past 2 decades in actual combat has resulted in its expansion to all military medical personnel as well as nonmedical special operators, conventional soldiers and Marines. Police SWAT medics, FBI Hostage Rescue Team, and so on, are also embracing its principles and adapting them to their situation.[20]

TCCC focuses on actions feasible for the medic under fire to improve the outcome of an injured soldier. A review of combat statistics has clearly illustrated that a significant proportion of fatalities were from hemorrhage, most frequently from the torso but also from the head, where there was little chance for control while actively engaging the enemy. However, approximately 20% of the KIA were from hemorrhage of an extremity, where there was a possibility of controlling the bleeding rapidly.[22,23] It is now accepted that causes of potentially preventable death ranked from most common to

Table 2
Definitions of the stages of tactical combat casualty care[21]

Stages of Care	
Care under fire	Care rendered by the combat medic or nonmedical combatant at the scene of injury while still under effective fire.
Tactical field care	Care rendered by the combat medic once no longer under effective hostile fire and also applies to situations where injury has occurred in the absence of hostile fire.
Tactical evacuation	Care rendered once the casualty has been transferred to an evacuation vehicle, that is, helicopter, armored vehicle, or ambulance.

From Butler, Jr FK, Hagmann J, Butler EG. Tactical combat casualty care in special operations. Mil Med 1996;161:3-16.

least, are (1) hemorrhage from a compressible site, (2) tension pneumothorax, and (3) airway compromise.

The first target was obtaining rapid control over extremity bleeding. Tourniquet use was sporadic in the Vietnam War, partly because of the conventional teaching that tourniquets were to be used only as a last resort and the issued or improvised tourniquets were frequently ineffective.[24] A better combat tourniquet was developed that could be self-applied with 1 hand by the injured combatant or medic. The current combat tourniquet has proven its worth and is now standard issue in medical personnel and combat troops' first aid kit.[25] For injuries that either are not amenable to a tourniquet or in addition to it, hemostatic agent-impregnated dressings have been developed and have been transitioned to the battlefield.[26] Under development are methods to transfuse blood products and administration of tranexamic acid pre-MTF, and the use of special clamp devices for hemorrhage of "junctional areas" (groin, neck, shoulder) and percutaneous intra-aortic balloon-tipped catheters for truncal hemorrhage.[27–30]

The second most common preventable cause of death is a tension pneumothorax, which has been attributed to an estimated 3% to 4% of all fatal injuries.[31] When suspected, the field expedient means of treatment remains needle thoracostomy. Once the casualty is at a BAS or Forward Resuscitative Surgical System or higher level of care, it can be converted to a thoracostomy tube with a negative-pressure collection device.

The third most frequent potentially survivable injury is the loss of airway. With an estimated 46% of fatal injuries involving the head and neck in the current conflicts, a compromised airway or need for airway protection is an obvious consideration.[22,23] However airway management other than the use of an nasopharyngeal or supraglottic airway paired with the "recovery" position are often the only practical actions that can be taken until the injured can be managed by more experienced medical personnel. Currently, the only maneuver taught to the battlefield medics is the emergency cricothyrotomy, as intubation is not a reliable option under combat conditions for a number of reasons.[32]

TACTICAL COMBAT CASUALTY CARE ACTIONS TAKEN IN EACH PHASE

The actions to be taken during each phase of TCCC are summarized here and in **Table 3**. Detailed current guidelines are available on-line and a review is recommended to better understand what care is likely to be provided before the anesthesiologist receives the patient.[33]

Table 3
Summary of tactical combat casualty care at each stage (2019)[33]

Stages of Care	Actions Taken
Care under fire	1. Return fire and take cover (casualty remains engaged if capable)
	2. Direct casualty if self-aid capable
	3. Protect casualty from further wounding
	4. Extract from burning vehicles or buildings and stop burning process
	5. Stop life-threatening external hemorrhage if tactically feasible
	6. Defer airway management until tactical field care phase
Tactical field care	1. Establish security perimeter
	2. Triage casualties, disarm those with altered mental status
	3. Reassess and treat unrecognized hemorrhage • Tourniquets • Hemostatic dressings • Bind pelvic fractures
	4. Airway management (recovery position, chin lift or jaw thrust, nasopharyngeal airway, supraglottic airway, or surgical cricothyrotomy)
	5. Assess and treat tension pneumothorax (needle thoracostomy)
	6. Assess and treat open or sucking chest wounds (vented chest seal)
	7. Obtain IV or IO access if in shock or impending shock • HepLock • Administer fluids if no-palpable pulses or unresponsive to voice • Hetastarch in normal saline (up to 1 L) if no blood products available and evidence of shock • Tranexamic acid if anticipate urgent blood transfusion and <3 h after wounding • If blood is available, whole blood or packed red blood cells, fresh frozen plasma, platelets in 1:1:1 ratio
	8. Hypothermia prevention
	9. Analgesia options (depends on shock state and level of consciousness) • TCCC Combat Wound Medication Pack (CWMP) - Tylenol 1300 mg PO Q8H, meloxicam 15 mg PO QD • Oral transmucosal fentanyl citrate 800 µg • Ketamine 50 mg IM or 20 mg IV • Morphine 5 mg IV
	10. Antibiotics options • Moxifloxacin 400 mg PO QD • Ertapenem 1 gm IV QD
	11. Burns: cover with dry sterile dressing, fluids per protocol, if available
	12. Fractures - splint, monitor peripheral pulses
	13. Communication • reassure casualty • arrange TACEVAC and prepare casualty for transport
	14. CPR is not reasonable on the battlefield unless situation rapidly reversed with bilateral needle thoracostomy
TACEVAC	1. Transition of care • Establish evacuation point security and stage casualties • Provide succinct hand off of care and TCCC Card documentation • TACEVAC medical personnel reassess casualties

(continued on next page)

Table 3 (continued)	
Stages of Care	**Actions Taken**
	2. TACEVAC plan of action is similar to tactical field care phase with the exception of available capabilities and expertise level of the TACEVAC crew
	3. Airway management: endotracheal intubation performed if required depending on tactical situation, available expertise, and equipment.
	4. Respiration • Monitor pulse oximetry • Supplementary O_2, if available for low SpO_2, unconscious, TBI, at altitude, and/or smoke inhalation
	5. Circulation • Vital signs monitoring, if available and tactical situation allows • Conversion of tourniquets to hemostatic or pressure dressings as soon as possible provided 3 criteria are met: (1) no shock present, (2) it is possible to monitor wound closely for rebleeding, (3) not controlling hemorrhage from traumatic amputation • Transfuse blood products if available and evidence of shock • Shock not responding to fluid resuscitation, repeat needle thoracostomy or if medical provider experience - tube thoracostomy
	6. CPR may be attempted if wounds not obviously fatal and will be arriving at surgical-capable MTF shortly

Abbreviations: CPR, cardiopulmonary resuscitation; IO, intraosseous; IV, intravenous; MTF, medical treatment facility; TACEVAC, tactical evacuation; TCCC, tactical combat casualty care; TBI, traumatic brain injury.

Data from Joint Trauma System. Tactical Combat Casualty Care Guidelines. Available at: https://jts.amedd.army.mil/assets/docs/cpgs/Prehospital_En_Route_CPGS/Tactical_Combat_Casualty_Care_Guidelines_01_Aug_2019. Accessed August 1, 2020.

Care under fire is very limited, as might be expected. The number one response of the responder is returning fire, including the casualty if capable, directing the casualty in self-aid if able, and protecting them from further injury. Depending on the circumstances, the casualty must be removed from any burning vehicle or building, the burning process suppressed, and any life-threatening external bleeding must be controlled. The application of tourniquets is appropriate if extremity arterial bleeding is evident. Airway management is really not feasible when actively engaged with the enemy. Once the casualties have been moved to a more secure site out of threat of direct fire, the combat medic or corpsman can initiate tactical field care actions.

In the tactical field care phase, perimeter security of the casualty collection site and tactical situation awareness must be maintained. Rapid triage of all casualties prioritizes the next set of actions. Obvious hemorrhage, new or renewed, is treated with either additional tourniquets or hemostatic-impregnated dressings and direct pressure. Compromised airways are addressed depending on the level of consciousness, with body position, jaw thrust maneuvers, nasopharyngeal airways, supraglottic airways (if available), or surgical cricothyrotomy if absolutely necessary. Open chest wounds are covered with a vented chest seal, and a suspected tension pneumothorax relieved with a needle thoracostomy. Endotracheal intubation is not undertaken in the tactical setting by combat medics owing to the lack of required experience and bulk of the necessary equipment.

A secondary patient assessment is conducted at this stage. Burns are addressed as feasible with dry sterile dressings and protocolized intravenous fluids if available.

Appreciate that, in the tactical setting, the combat medic is limited by what can be physically carried or stored in the limited space of a mounted patrol vehicle. Intravenous or intraosseous (usually sternum) access is obtained, but flushed and locked. Fluid administration, generally limited to colloid (500 mL bags), is only administered to patients in shock. Shock at this stage is assessed clinically by mental state, peripheral pulses, and perhaps by finger pulse oximetry. Antibiotics and analgesics are administered as required and available, the latter sparingly depending on hemodynamic and mental status. All fractures are stabilized to prevent further neurovascular injury and pain. Finally, casualty evacuation must be arranged by helicopter, ambulance, or armored combat vehicle of opportunity. The tactical situation (active or controlled), suitability of landing zones or route, and distance to the MTF often dictates the plan.

The TACEVAC phase in general follows the same treatment plans, with the main exceptions being the TACEVAC platform, the additional supplies and equipment provided, and the overall expertise and experience level of the medical team. TACEVAC is a general term combining the terms CASEVAC (the evacuation of casualties from the point of wounding, which can be still be involved in hostile action) and MEDEVAC (the transport of casualties between one medical facility which can be a Role 1 BAS or Shock Trauma Platoon, to a higher level MTF). During the conflicts in Iraq and Afghanistan, various platforms were used and requirements changed as the theater matured and Role 2 and 3 MTFs were established throughout the country. Even so, helicopters remained the most commonly used mode of expedient transport. In Iraq, the dedicated Army HH-60M Blackhawk air ambulance was most frequently used for MEDEVAC and CASEVAC within theater, could transport up to 6 litters on special stanchions with 1 flight medic on board, and has on-board O_2 generator capability. Other services often used aircraft of opportunity with their own medical support on board.

Special Operations Forces (SOF) frequently used helicopters already engaged in supporting their assaults and capable of landing in confined landing zones. Therefore, the mission profile always included at least one medical provider on-board one helicopter to provide advanced monitoring and advanced trauma life support capability (JMJ personal communication). On an HH-60H Seahawk (SOF variant), space was limited to 2 floor-loaded patients and 1 sitting casualty because 2 door gunners share the space with their mounted machine guns and boxes of ammunition. Because all missions were conducted at night using night vision goggles, strict light discipline was observed and all patient assessment decreased to palpation and search for wounds, verbal challenge, and a cloaked electronic monitor if applied. If any additional invasive procedures were required en route, they were performed undercover to minimize any light signature. In more open rural Iraq, SOF used the larger USAF MH-53 Pavelow helicopter with either their Special Tactics PJs or Special Operations Medical Element (SOFME = SOF flight surgeon plus 1–2 Independent Duty Medical Technicians) on board poised in a quick reaction response mode. They were capable of carrying 20 casualties and considerable advanced trauma life support supplies, including a portable blood refrigerator.

In Afghanistan, a wide variety of helicopters were used in the CASEVAC role, but given the mountainous terrain and associated power requirements, the powerful Army MH-47 Chinook helicopter or tilt-rotor V-22 Osprey is used most frequently. The larger aircraft can accommodate up to 20 litters on the floor and include a USA or USAF Special Operations medical team on board. Their average transit times to a Role 2 MTF are considerably longer than those in Iraq.

CASUALTY CARE AT IN-THEATER ROLE 2 AND ROLE 3 TREATMENT FACILITIES AND BEYOND

The golden hour remains a guiding principle in trauma care and wounded combatants are rapidly transported from the BAS or battlefield to the nearest higher level of care—a Role 2 or Role 3 facility—depending on the nature and severity of injury. The Role 2 MTF can be a USA Forward Surgical Team, a USN Forward Resuscitative Surgical System, or a USAF Expeditionary Medical Support, occupying a mobile tent hospital or an established permanent structure. Staffing typically includes emergency medicine physicians; general, trauma, and/or orthopedic surgeons; anesthesiologists; certified registered nurse anesthetists; physician assistants; nursing staff; and hospital corpsman and medics. Capability includes a limited emergency department and operating rooms for damage control resuscitation and surgery, and limited in-patient beds primarily for brief surgical recovery before MEDEVAC or those that can be returned to duty. Ancillary services may include laboratory and radiologic services (plain film, ultrasound machine, and the occasional computed tomography scanner), and blood products may be obtained from a limited supply of stored blood or via emergency blood donation from the "walking blood bank." Upon activation, service members with type O blood quickly report to the medical facility to donate. From the time of donation and screening, transfusion into the injured patient usually occurs in 30 to 45 minutes, and patients receive whole blood. At this level of care, the goal of patient care is rapid triage, surgical stabilization and salvage, and MEDEVAC to a higher echelon of care in less than 24 hours, with the most acute patients receiving the highest priority for transport.

Role 3 facilities are the highest level of medical care available within a combat zone. Examples include USA Combat Support Hospitals, USAF Theater Hospitals, Regional Trauma Hospitals (such as the Kandahar Air Field Role 3 Multinational Medical Unit in Afghanistan), Fleet Hospitals, and Hospital Ships, for example, the USNS Mercy and USNS Comfort. These facilities offer support from a multitude of surgical and medical specialties and have a more robust capability for inpatient and rehabilitative care, but supplies can sometimes be limited and unpredictable (**Table 4**). At this level, care remains focused on damage control resuscitation and "life-, limb-, or eyesight-"saving surgery with further MEDEVAC anticipated.[13–18] If evacuation is delayed, more extensive surgical repairs and washouts may be possible, although the ultimate goal is expedited patient movement to the continental US health care system.

PATIENT CARE CONSIDERATIONS FROM THE POINT OF INJURY

From the point of injury, CASEVAC to the nearest Role 2 or 3 facility via helicopter is most common (**Fig. 1**). While en route, radio communication with the receiving facility involves the use of a "9-Line" report, which includes the number, nationality, and type and severity of injuries. Upon arrival, patients are screened for the presence of firearms or explosive devices and retriaged (**Fig. 2**). Even US and coalition, or "friendly," forces are disarmed because they may become disoriented and confuse medical staff as hostile combatants.

As described elsewhere in this article, injuries from explosives frequently require tourniquets and/or pelvic binders to control bleeding and yet may have lost an excessive amount of blood. They arrive "alive but empty." Therefore the treatment of hypoperfusion, and the potential lethal triad of acidosis, hypothermia, and coagulopathy, as well as the accompanying traumatic shock, is paramount. There is a 4-fold increase in mortality if left unchecked.[12–14]

Table 4
Role 3 MTF clinical staffing

Surgical Services	#	Nonsurgical Services	#
Trauma surgery	1	Adult/pediatric critical care	2
General surgery	3	Internal medicine	1
Orthopedic Surgery	3	Emergency medicine	5
Oromaxillofacial surgery	1	Family medicine	3
Neurosurgery	1	Neurology	1
Ophthalmology	1	Radiology	1
OB/Gyn	1	Interventional radiology	1
Anesthesiology/CRNA	6	Mental health	5
Orthopedic PA	1	Optometry	1
		Social work	1
		Dental	2

Upon arrival at the Role 2 or 3 unit, trauma care follows the team-based advanced trauma life support principles. In the trauma bay, assessment begins with the primary and secondary surveys; stabilizing life-threatening insults to circulation, airway, and breathing; and identifying all potential injuries. Members of the trauma team are strategically staged around the patient with the anesthesiologist at the head of the bed. Monitors are placed and peripheral or central intravenous, or intraosseous, access is secured. If a definitive airway is required, gentle rapid sequence induction with in-line cervical stabilization is usually performed using etomidate, propofol, or ketamine and succinylcholine, vecuronium, or rocuronium with or without adjuncts such as fentanyl or lidocaine, and often with simultaneous volume resuscitation. Trauma-induced hypotension is generally owing to hypovolemia so vasopressors should be used as a temporizing measure or avoided if possible. Likewise, overcorrection of blood

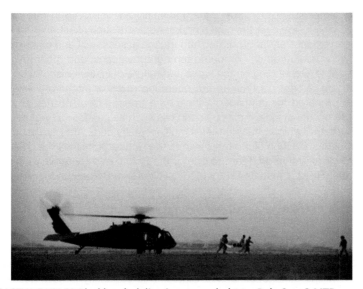

Fig. 1. CASEVAC HH-60 Blackhawk delivering wounded to a Role 2 or 3 MTF.

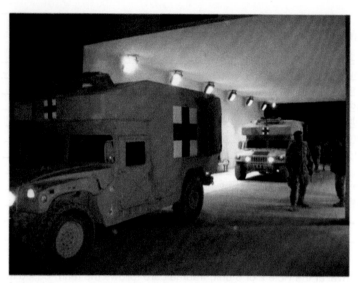

Fig. 2. Ambulance bay at a Role 3 MTF, Afghanistan. Multiple combat casualties transported from adjoining airfield undergoing triage and dis-arming.

pressure should be avoided. The target is a mean arterial pressure of greater than 55 mm Hg or a systolic blood pressure of greater than 90 mm Hg, which has been demonstrated to improve survival. A rapid infusing device such as the Belmont is used for the rapid transfusion of warmed packed red blood cells to plasma to platelets at a 1:1:1 ratio. During transfusion, care is taken to avoid hypocalcemia and hyperkalemia. For refractory hypotension, and despite aggressive volume resuscitation, a trial of vasopressor (such as vasopressin as an intravenous bolus or infusion), and hydrocortisone 100 mg intravenously, may be considered. In the past, recombinant factor VII was used to treat refractory bleeding, but has fallen out of favor. Tranexamic acid is now a mainstay of treatment and is usually administered in the trauma bay and followed by infusion over the next 8 hours. Adjuncts such as ultrasound examination have been extensively incorporated into trauma assessment and management, as well as plain film radiography, computed tomography scans, and other ancillary services as available. Depending on the types and nature of injuries discovered, resuscitation and management continue in the operating room or intensive care unit, and patients are prepared for continued critical care transport out of theater. The next phase of care occurs at Role 4 military hospitals such as Landstuhl Regional Medical Center in Germany, which offer high-level multispecialty care. After further evaluation and care, patients are then ultimately flown to the United States via the USAF Critical Care Aeromedical Transport Team to one of the Role 5 military tertiary care centers such as Walter Reed National Military Medical Center in Bethesda, Maryland.

CRITICAL CARE AEROMEDICAL TRANSPORT TEAM

Early in the 1990s, the USAF expanded its aeromedical capabilities to the point of providing fairly sophisticated critical care to patients during prolonged transports (MEDEVAC) from the theater of operations to external MTFs, for example, Europe, and then on to the continental United States. This capability is now referred to as the Critical Care Aeromedical Transport Team. As an emphasis on early evacuation has grown, freshly stabilized casualties following damage control surgery may be transported within 24 to 48 hours of wounding and surgery to distant MTFs for definitive surgery.

CRITICAL CARE AEROMEDICAL TRANSPORT TEAM COMPOSITION

The standard Critical Care Aeromedical Transport Team consists of a physician with a background in critical care from anesthesiology, emergency medicine, pulmonary critical care, or trauma surgery, a registered nurse with at least 2 years of experience in critical care, and a certified respiratory therapist. In addition to qualifying in their specialty and critical care, all members undergo 2 to 4 weeks of additional training involving simulation, didactics, and hands-on cadaveric skills specifically addressing a wide array of topics, including altitude and hyperbaric physiology, burn wound management, mechanical ventilation of acute respiratory distress syndrome using transport ventilators, spine precautions, management of elevated intracranial pressure in flight, extracorporeal membrane oxygenation, and more. All members must be physically qualified for flight status.

Additionally, an Acute Lung Rescue Team (ALRT) has been formed to transport those patients requiring extracorporeal life support systems. This team is composed of the same members as the Critical Care Aeromedical Transport Team, with the addition of a critical care surgeon and an additional critical care nurse and respiratory therapist.

PATIENT SELECTION AND PREPARATION

These transports can be performed in many types of USAF aircraft but most frequently used are the C-130 and C-17 carrying between 74 and 90 casualties, depending on the aircraft and patient severity, and can last 8 to 10 hours or longer and cover thousands of miles before arriving at the MTF (**Fig. 3**). Therefore, many patient

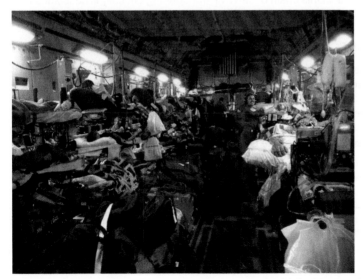

Fig. 3. A Critical Care Aeromedical Transport Team evacuating multiple OEF casualties from Germany to United States hospitals in a C-17. Note the stanchions inserted in the cargo bay enable "stacking" up to 3 litters.

considerations must be addressed before flying with combat casualty, including the effects of altitude physiology on their specific injuries and general physical condition, oxygen requirements and supplies, the flight environment, and even the mission needs. Altitude physiology can affect every organ system: from the head to the heart, kidneys, and even the gastrointestinal tract. Abnormal heart rhythms and other cardiac pathologies are something to strongly consider, especially those with chest trauma. For those patients with pulmonary injury including contusions, rib fractures, hemo-thorax or pneumothorax, acute respiratory distress syndrome with increasing Fio_2 and positive end-expiratory pressure requirements, pneumonia, or even those patients with high opioid requirements, could put the patient at risk for respiratory depression, which must be mitigated.

Critical Care Aeromedical Transport Teams are designed to be flexible and highly mobile in response to emergency missions and operate across the spectrum of potential scenarios from humanitarian relief operations to major theaters of war. Equipment for patient transport needs to be reliable, durable, with adequate battery life, and compatible with flight operations (vibration, pressure changes, electrical or radio interference). Despite these many challenges, CCAT teams are able to transport large numbers of patients including those requiring continued stabilization en route.

SUMMARY

The practice of medicine (anesthesiology and critical care) in a deployed combat setting requires a wide range of medical skills and knowledge, creativity, adaptability, and resilience to enable continuous performance under duress. The US Military Joint Trauma System has been successful in mitigating the impact of these harsh conditions under which care for the combat casualty is provided and establishes continuity of care from the battlefield to US medical centers. Its components were briefly reviewed with emphasis on combat trauma care under fire and the role of the anesthesiologist in this continuum of care. The USAF Critical Care Aeromedical Transport Team is an important link in this chain of survival, transporting critically ill casualties from the theater to higher levels of care outside the war zone and home.

DISCLOSURE

The views expressed in this article reflect the results of research conducted by the author(s) and do not necessarily reflect the official policy or position of the Department of the Navy or the Air Force, Department of Defense, Department of Veterans Affairs Administration, nor the United States Government.

Darian Rice is a military service member and Brooke Albright-Trainer is a federal/contracted employee of the United States government.

CLINICS CARE POINTS

- Combat produces horrific injuries in large numbers quickly and treatment begins on the battlefield.
- Survivable injuries require immediate attention to control bleeding and address respiratory compromise even while under hostile fire.
- The Joint Trauma System is a proven concept providing the right amount of care as far forward as possible and evacuating the patient to staged higher levels of care quickly and efficiently.

- The anesthesiologist/intensivist plays a crucial role in nearly every stage and requires a high degree of focus, skill, tenacity, and adaptability to perform well.
- The Critical Care Aeromedical Transport Team is an integral part of the Joint Trauma System and ensures continuity of critical care for the combat casualty as they progress through this system.

REFERENCES

1. Holcomb JB, Stansbury LG, Champion HR, et al. Understanding combat casualty care statistics. J Trauma 2006;60:397–401.
2. Eastridge BJ, Mabry RL, Seguin P, et al. Death on the battlefield (2001-2011): implications for the future of combat casualty care. J Trauma Acute Care Surg 2012; 73:S431–7.
3. Howard JT, Kotwal RS, Stern CA, et al. Use of combat casualty care data to assess the US Military Trauma System during the Afghanistan and Iraq conflicts, 2001-2017. JAMA Surg 2019;154(7):600–8.
4. Le TD, Gurney JM, Nnamani NS, et al. A 12-year analysis of nonbattle injury among US service member deployed to Iraq and Afghanistan. JAMA Surg 2018;153(9):800–7.
5. Owens BD, Kragh JF, Wenke JC, et al. Combat wounds in Operation Iraqi Freedom and Operations Enduring Freedom. J Trauma 2008;64:295–9.
6. Champion HR, Holcomb JB, Young LA. Injuries from explosions: physics, biophysics, pathology, and required research focus. J Trauma 2009;66:1468–77.
7. Ritenour AE, Blackbourne LH, Kelly JF, et al. Incidence of primary blast injury in US military overseas contingency operations. Ann Surg 2010;251:1140–4.
8. Stefanopoulos PK, Mikros G, Pinialidis DE, et al. Wound ballistics of military rifle bullets: an update on controversial issues and associated misconceptions. J Trauma Acute Care Surg 2019;87(3):690–8.
9. Maiden N. Ballistics reviews: mechanisms of bullet wound trauma. Forensic Sci Med Pathol 2009;5:204–9.
10. Artz CP, Bronwell AW, Sako Y. Experiences in the management of abdominal and thoracoabdominal injuries in Korea. Am J Surg 1955;89(4):773–9.
11. Cohen MJ, West M. Acute traumatic coagulopathy: from endogenous acute coagulopathy to systemic acquired coagulopathy and back. J Trauma 2011;70(5 Suppl):S47–9.
12. Cannon JW. Hemorrhagic shock. N Engl J Med 2018;178(4):370–9.
13. Shapiro MB, Jenkins DH, Schwab CW, et al. Damage control: collective review. J Trauma 2000;49:969–78.
14. U.S. Military Joint Trauma System. Damage control resuscitation. Available at: https://jts.amedd.army.mil/assets/docs/cpgs/JTS_Clinical_Practice_Guidelines_ (CPGS)/Damage_Control_Resuscitation_12_Jul_2019_ID18. Accessed August 6, 2020.
15. Rotondo MF, Schwab CW, McGonigal MD, et al. 'Damage control': an approach for improved survival in exsanguinating penetrating abdominal injury. J Trauma 1993;35(3):375–82.
16. Cotton BA, Guy JS, Morris JA Jr, et al. The cellular, metabolic, and systemic consequences of aggressive fluid resuscitation strategies. Shock 2006;26(2):115–21.
17. Cotton BA, Reddy N, Hatch QM, et al. Damage control resuscitation is associated with a reduction in resuscitation volumes and improvement in survival in 390 damage control laparotomy patients. Ann Surg 2011;254(4):598–605.

18. Blackbourne LH. Combat damage control surgery. Crit Care Med 2008; 36(Suppl):S304–10.
19. Bagg MR, Covey DC, Powell ET. Levels of medical care in the Global War on Terrorism. J Am Acad Orthop Surg 2006;14:S7–9.
20. Butler FK Jr. Tactical Combat Casualty Care: beginnings. Wilderness Environ Med 2017;28:S12–7.
21. Butler FK Jr, Hagmann J, Butler EG. Tactical combat casualty care in special operations. Mil Med 1996;161:3–16.
22. Champion HR, Bellamy RF, Roberts P, et al. A profile of combat injury. J Trauma 2003;54(5):S13–9.
23. Eastridge BJ, Hardin M, Cantrell J, et al. Died of wounds on the battlefield: causation and implications for improving combat casualty care. J Trauma 2011; 71(1):S4–8.
24. Kragh JF, Swan KG, Smith DC, et al. Historical review of emergency tourniquet use to stop bleeding. Am J Surg 2012;203:242–52.
25. Kragh JF, Walters TJ, Baer DG, et al. Survival with emergency tourniquet use to stop bleeding in major limb trauma. Ann Surg 2009;249:1–7.
26. Tompeck AJ, Gajdhar AR, Dowling M, et al. A comprehensive review of topical hemostatic agents: the good, the bad, and the novel. J Trauma Acute Care Surg 2020;88:e1–21.
27. Mabry RL, McManus JG. Prehospital advances in the management of severe penetrating trauma. Crit Care Med 2008;36(Suppl):S528–66.
28. Shackelford SA, del Junco DJ, Powel–Dunford N, et al. Association of prehospital blood product transfusion during medical evacuation of combat casualties in Afghanistan with acute and 30-day survival. JAMA 2017;318(16):1581–91.
29. Huebner BR, Dorlac WC, Cribari C. Tranexamic acid use in prehospital uncontrolled hemorrhage. Wilderness Environ Med 2017;28:S50–60.
30. Martin MJ, Holcomb JB, Polk T, et al. The "top 10" research and development priorities for battlefield surgical care: results from the Committee on Surgical Combat Casualty Care research gap analysis. J Trauma Acute Care Surg 2019; 87(Suppl 1):S14–21.
31. McPherson JJ, Feigin DS, Bellamy RF. Prevalence of tension pneumothorax in fatally wounded combat casualties. J Trauma 2006;60:573–8.
32. Mabry RL, Kharod CU, Bennett BL. Awake cricothyrotomy: a novel approach to the surgical airway in the tactical setting. Wilderness Environ Med 2017;28: S61–8.
33. Joint Trauma System. Tactical combat casualty care guidelines. Available at: https://jts.amedd.army.mil/assets/docs/cpgs/Prehospital_En_Route_CPGS/ Tactical_Combat_Casualty_Care_Guidelines_01_Aug_2019. Accessed August 1, 2020.
34. Pruitt BA Jr. Combat casualty and surgical progress. Ann Surg 2006;243(6): 715–29.

Regional Anesthesia in the Field for Trauma Victims

Robert Vietor III, MD*, Chester Buckenmaier III, MS, MD

KEYWORDS

- Regional • Anesthesia • Trauma • Disaster • Nerve • Austere • Field • Block

KEY POINTS

- Anesthesiologists can provide regional anesthesia techniques to relieve pain, facilitate surgical procedures, and are crucial to patient care in field environments.
- Regional anesthesia offers several advantages over general anesthesia in field environments.
- Because of the decrease in risks associated with ultrasound-guided blocks compared with landmark techniques with nerve stimulation, ultrasound is the preferred method for most blocks in field environments.
- Creating a pain management system to follow patients from point of injury to definitive care is important when performing regional anesthesia in the field.
- Regional anesthesia is only one aspect of multimodal pain management.

INTRODUCTION

Anesthesiologists have an important role in the care of trauma patients in the field, especially in times of disaster. The field encompasses environments where medical facilities are unavailable or when arrival at facilities will be delayed. Regional anesthesia has emerged as a technique provided by anesthesiologists that can have a major impact in managing pain following trauma and surgery and moderate the need for general anesthetics in austere environments. When considering regional anesthesia for patients in field environments, it is important to adequately prepare for anticipated patients, mitigate risks, and understand the advantages of regional anesthesia in resource-challenged conditions.

Discussion

Preparation

Preparing for anticipated patients is critical. Preparation includes assessing the patient population at risk, the traumatic injuries most likely to occur, and the resources

The authors have nothing to disclose. The views presented here do not represent the views of the US Military, the Department of Defense or the Uniformed Services University.
Anesthesiology, Uniformed Services University, 4301 Jones Bridge Road, Bethesda, MD 20814, USA
* Corresponding author.
E-mail address: ROBERT.VIETOR@USUHS.EDU

Anesthesiology Clin 39 (2021) 337–351
https://doi.org/10.1016/j.anclin.2021.02.006
1932-2275/21/Published by Elsevier Inc.

available. During times of disaster, the affected populations can vary greatly, and clinicians who typically care for adult trauma patients may find themselves caring for large populations of children, pregnant women, or elderly depending on the situation. Much of the equipment required for regional anesthesia is similar across these populations, which enhances the value of regional anesthesia as an option for a wide range of patients compared with general anesthesia. Studies show that more than 40% of trauma patients sustain extremity injuries.[1,2] Patients with extremity injuries are good candidates for regional anesthesia and often undergo procedures using only a regional anesthetic. Obviously, regional anesthesia will not meet all anesthesia needs in field environments, but effective utilization of regional anesthesia preserves available resources and helps avoid general anesthetics.

In addition to supplies required to perform regional anesthesia in the field, it is important to have emergency equipment associated with regional and general anesthesia. Every situation is unique but when possible standard ASA monitors, lipid emulsion, emergency airway devices, and cardiovascular medications should be available.[3] In field environments, the ability to care for patients with minimal supplies and manpower is critical, and the effective use of regional anesthesia helps make this possible.

In addition to preparing to perform regional anesthesia techniques in field environments, it is also important to have a care system in place from the point of injury to definitive care. This comprehensive care system for regional anesthesia requires specialized, coordinated care from anesthesiologists, and other health care providers. An example of this is the US military's system that was established in the early 2000s. In 2003, during the war in Iraq, the first continuous peripheral nerve catheter for a battlefield injury was placed.[4] Since then regional anesthesia, especially continuous peripheral nerve catheters, have become commonplace for casualties injured on the battlefield being transported back to definitive care in both the United States and other allied nations.[5,6] The adoption of regional anesthesia and peripheral nerve catheters in war casualties was due in part to the failure of opioid reliant strategies for pain control and the complications that are associated with those strategies.[6]

To address issues associated with opioids, the Army Regional Anesthesia and Pain Management Initiative was established and promoted multimodal and regional anesthesia techniques in war wounded.[7] Soon after, the Military Advanced Regional Anesthesia and Analgesia group encouraged coordination with all branches of the US armed forces.[8] Several successful acute pain services were established in field environments such as Camp Bastion in Afghanistan.[9] Although the establishment of an acute pain service in the field can provide the initial pain control and catheter placement for these patients, it is important to continue the comprehensive pain management as the patient is evacuated to definitive care.

Carness and colleagues[10] looked at aeromedical evacuation patients leaving Bagram airfield in Afghanistan, traveling to Landstuhl Regional Medical Center and then to the continental United States from 2009 to 2013. They found that the average time from Bagram to the United States was 5.26 days, yet 38% of the patients had their continuous peripheral nerve catheters removed.[10] Although some of these catheters were removed for good reason, many of the reasons for catheter removal were not recorded in the patient record.[10] Given the benefits of catheters in these patients, it is crucial that functioning catheters remain in place during the evacuation process. When catheters are removed, strong consideration should be given to replacing them when clinically appropriate. To avoid the inappropriate discontinuation of continuous peripheral nerve catheters, providers caring for these patients along the evacuation route must be well trained in pain management and catheter management and educated in the benefits of regional anesthesia for trauma patients.

Advantages of regional anesthesia

Advantages of regional anesthesia techniques, when compared with general anesthesia in field environments, include alleviating patient pain while preserving general function, decreased resource utilization, and general improved recovery. One major advantage is the ability to treat pain or perform procedures while preserving patient consciousness and physical function. This is beneficial when trauma victims have injuries that are amenable to regional anesthesia but still need to make decisions, perform manual tasks, or require the ability to move to another location.

Regional anesthesia techniques anesthetize only a region of the body; thus a patient may lose function of one extremity but can still maintain the use of other extremities. Perhaps more importantly, the preservation of patient cognition allows them to actively participate in their evacuation to higher levels of care. Contrast this with a general anesthetic where the patient will not only be unable to function but will require additional care team members to transport and care for the patient. Systemic medications used for pain relief and general anesthesia will decease a patient's cognitive and physical abilities, which can be dangerous in field environments. Regional anesthesia also decreases the amount of opioids consumed by surgical patients.[11] US military efforts in regional anesthesia techniques during the wars in Iraq and Afghanistan have shown that patients receiving continuous nerve block catheters report less pain than those without, and as a result they experience decreased anxiety, worry, and distress during transport.[12] In addition, regional anesthesia has been shown to decrease chronic pain in patients undergoing surgery and may decrease the chance of patients developing complex regional pain syndrome.[13,14] Another advantage of regional anesthesia is the utilization of fewer resources to perform a regional anesthetic. With the exception of ultrasonography, many regional anesthetics can be performed with supplies that are readily available such as needles, syringes, and local anesthetics. A general anesthetic requires additional medications, which may be difficult to obtain, carry, and store in field environments. Many general anesthetics will also require a method to provide positive pressure ventilation and more labor intensive intra- and postoperative care.

For these reasons, military forward surgical units use regional anesthetics at much higher rates when compared with civilian medical facilities.[15] Finally, many regional techniques are simple to perform compared with a general anesthetic. Single injection nerve blocks can be performed in a few minutes and provide hours of relief of patient pain. With the placement of continuous nerve catheters, the analgesia can safely be extended for days or weeks.[16,17] All of these advantages make regional anesthesia a superior option to general anesthesia for many situations in the field.

Risks of regional anesthesia

In field environments, similar to the hospital environment, mitigating risks such as injection site infections, local anesthetic toxicity, and bleeding complications is important. One risk that is present in both environments is procedure site infections. Aseptic technique should always be used when performing regional anesthesia.[18] Interestingly, despite difficulties of cleanliness in field environments, infection does not seem to be a significant issue for regional techniques performed in field environments. During the Iraq War from 2003 to 2004, infection rates in evacuated causalities with indwelling catheters was found to be 1.9%.[17] Compare this with catheters performed in ideal conditions, where one study found an overall incidence of catheter-related infections around 2.9%.[19] These rates suggest that although care should be taken to avoid catheter-related infections, the placement of peripheral nerve catheters in the field is safe. This same study found that the incidence of infections in ideal conditions started to increase at catheter day 4[19]; this supports a case series that noted that the most significant factor in their facility's catheter site infections in combat-related injuries was duration of catheter use.[20]

Similar to other indwelling devices, it is important to assess continuous peripheral nerve catheters daily for signs of infection.[21] It is also prudent to remove continuous peripheral nerve catheters as soon as it is clinically reasonable. The decision to remove a catheter requires anesthesiologists to assess a patient's pain management needs and clinical picture.[21] Fortunately, most catheter site infections are easily treated with catheter removal and possibly antibiotics. Catheter site infections requiring surgical intervention are rare and occur in 0.9% of catheter infections.[21]

A second risk is local anesthetic systemic toxicity (LAST). LAST is always a concern when performing regional anesthesia. The treatment of LAST can be resource intensive, time consuming, and may result in poor outcomes for the patient. Therefore, avoidance of LAST is of the utmost importance. Using ultrasound over landmark and nerve stimulation techniques for regional anesthesia may help avoid LAST.[22] Although many regional anesthetic techniques can be successfully performed using landmark techniques and nerve stimulation, advances in ultrasound have significantly improved the safety and success rates of regional anesthesia. Bomberg and colleagues[23] found that vascular puncture occurred in 0.9% of patients receiving peripheral nerve blocks with ultrasound and 2.4% of patients receiving peripheral nerve blocks with landmarks and nerve stimulation. Given the catastrophic consequences of an intravascular injection while performing a peripheral nerve block in field environments, it is recommended that ultrasound be used for regional anesthesia whenever it is available. In addition, ultrasound-guided nerve blocks are associated with increased rates of success when compared with other methods of performance.[24]

Modern ultrasound equipment is easy to transport to out-of-hospital locations and has been used in field environments by the US military for the last 2 decades.[25] The cost of ultrasound has decreased significantly over the same time. In instances where ultrasound is not available, landmark approaches with nerve stimulation can still be used while being mindful of the risks associated with such procedures and the resources available to treat complications. Peripheral nerve stimulation techniques have safely been used in regional anesthesia for decades and provide an indispensable backup to ultrasonography for anesthesiologists providing care in field environments. Nerve stimulation may also be useful when there is difficulty visualizing a nerve with ultrasound or when the cost of a modern ultrasound machine is prohibitive.[26]

Finally, bleeding complications require special considerations in field environments. In many field environments, coagulation studies may not be available; therefore, a good patient history to assess for bleeding risk is important. In addition, should a patient develop a hematoma, treatment of the hematoma, such as platelets or surgical intervention, may not be available. These complications, and the ability to treat them, should be considered when choosing regional anesthesia techniques and procedures that are appropriate for a particular situation. By mitigating the risks associated with regional anesthesia in field environments, anesthesiologists can safely provide patients with pain relief and an alternative to general anesthesia for surgical procedures.

Regional techniques frequently used in the field

There are many regional techniques that are beneficial for trauma patients in field environments. After taking into account the injuries frequently seen in trauma patients, the benefits of regional anesthesia, and the risks of regional anesthesia in the field, many of the peripheral nerve block techniques that offer the most benefit with a reasonable amount of risk are of the upper and lower extremities. At a minimum, anesthesiologists should be familiar with the unique indications, risks, and benefits of the following regional techniques when providing care in field environments. There are many sources that can be referenced to provide detailed descriptions for the performance of these regional techniques.[8,27]

Upper extremity

Digital nerve blocks Digital nerve blocks are useful for laceration repair or surgical procedures involving the digits. The digital nerves travel along the volar aspect of both sides of the digit. There are several techniques that are used for digital nerve blocks. The most efficient, yet effective technique for the digital nerve block is a single subcutaneous injection on the volar surface of the digit at the metacarpal phalangeal joint.[28] Of note, a similar injection at the proximal interphalangeal joint is effective for fingertip injuries and produces faster onset of anesthesia.[29] The use of epinephrine to extend the duration of digital blocks is controversial, and despite some studies suggesting that it is safe,[30] epinephrine should not be used for digital blocks. There are long-acting local anesthetics that do not risk digital ischemia. For example, using bupivacaine for digital block has been shown to have a 15-hour duration of analgesia.[31] Finally, compartment syndrome can develop whenever there is an increase in the contents of the compartment without an appropriate increase in the myofascial envelope.[32] Therefore, injecting a large volume of local anesthetic into the fixed space of the finger may lead to ischemia or compartment syndrome. The proceduralist should use only enough volume to accomplish the block and be aware of patient complaints of pain or resistance to injection of local anesthetic.

Individual nerve blocks of the arm Regional techniques of individual nerves of the forearm are useful for larger hand and forearm injuries. The ulnar, radial, and median nerves can all be targeted for pain relief of injuries and analgesia during procedures. All 3 of these blocks are used for laceration repair, abscess drainage, and foreign body removal within their respective areas of sensory innervation.[33] The ulnar nerve typically provides cutaneous sensory innervation to half of the fourth digit, the entire fifth digit, and the ulnar aspect of the hand.[34] Ulnar nerve blocks can be used to treat pain or facilitate surgery related to fifth digit injuries such as boxer fractures.[35] The radial nerve typically provides sensory innervation to the dorsum of the hand.[36] A supracondylar radial nerve block can successfully treat pain from a distal radial fracture and allow reduction of the fracture without sedation.[37] The median nerve provides sensory innervation to the palm of the hand—the first, second, third, and half of the fourth digit.[38] Median nerve blocks can help relieve pain from fractures in the first 3 digits of the hand. All 3 nerves of the forearm can be performed with few materials, and regional techniques can be performed at multiple locations along the nerves based on the patient's site of injury. Of note, all of the nerves of the forearm can be located under ultrasound in relation to the axillary artery in the upper arm and blocked together or followed down the arm to allow regional anesthesia techniques of these individual nerves above the elbow. When blocking these nerves near the axillary artery an ultrasound approach is preferred, but it is important to remember that a transaxillary artery approach can be used to block the ulnar, radial, and median nerves if ultrasound is not available. When performing all forearm nerve blocks, make note to avoid the colocated arteries. Given the close proximity of the axillary artery to the nerves in the axilla, avoiding intravascular injection is important for these regional anesthesia techniques. Consider blocking the musculocutaneous nerve when anesthesia on the volar side of the skin below the elbow is required.[39]

Supraclavicular brachial plexus nerve block The supraclavicular brachial plexus nerve block is useful for surgical procedures and pain in the upper extremity below the shoulder and axilla to include fractures, dislocations, and abscesses (**Fig. 1**). Stone and colleagues[40] found that ultrasound-guided regional anesthesia of the brachial plexus decreased emergency department length of stay compared with procedural sedation. In field environments, decreasing recovery times can be crucial. Ultrasonography has significantly decreased complications associated with supraclavicular brachial plexus blocks. Pneumothorax is a known complication of the supraclavicular brachial plexus block. When conducting periclavicular blocks, the incidence of pneumothorax without the use of ultrasound was found to be as high 6.1%, whereas using ultrasound the incidence was 0.06%.[41] A second common complication of the supraclavicular brachial plexus block is phrenic nerve paralysis, which has been shown to occur in up to 60% of patients receiving a block.[42] Because of the proximity of the brachial plexus to the subclavian artery, care must be taken to avoid intravascular injection.

Interscalene brachial plexus nerve block The interscalene brachial plexus nerve block is useful for surgical procedures on the shoulder. One unique indication for this block in the field is the reduction of shoulder dislocations.[43] There is some evidence that prehospital ultrasound-guided interscalene blocks may actually improve the ability to reduce shoulder dislocations compared with other methods of pain

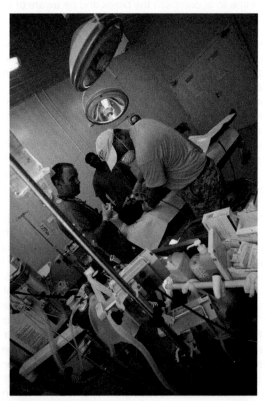

Fig. 1. Administering a supraclavicular block for surgery on an injured Iraqi national for right extremity trauma.

control and sedation.[44] To perform this block, local anesthetic should be injected where the brachial plexus travels between the anterior and middle scalene muscles. A common complication of the interscalene brachial plexus block is phrenic nerve paralysis, which, depending on technique, has been shown to occur in up to 100% of patients receiving the block.[45] A few studies have shown that lower doses of local anesthetic may decrease phrenic nerve paralysis while providing similar analgesia for patients.[46] Therefore, ultrasound guidance and low-dose blocks may be beneficial in patients who may not tolerate phrenic nerve paralysis well. An additional complication that is rarely seen is spinal anesthesia following interscalene brachial plexus block.[47]

Lower extremity

Ankle block The ankle block is useful for surgery or pain involving the foot and digits of the foot. Typically, 5 nerves are blocked with this regional technique. Four of the nerves originate with the sciatic nerve and include the posterior tibial nerve, the deep peroneal nerve, the superficial peroneal nerve, and the sural nerve. The fifth nerve is the saphenous nerve, which is a branch of the femoral nerve.[48] Although it is common for the ankle block to be performed based solely on anatomic landmarks, Chin and colleagues[49] revealed that ankle blocks performed under ultrasound guidance were more successful in achieving adequate surgical anesthesia. In their study they used a combination of ultrasound and anatomic landmarks in the ultrasound group due to the difficulty in locating smaller nerves on ultrasound; this is possibly due to anatomic variation in the location and innervation of the nerves of the foot and ankle.

The posterior tibial nerve provides sensation to the mid- and forefoot bony structures and the skin of the plantar foot and travels posterior and superficial to the medial malleolus. It is located near the posterior tibial artery at the ankle.[50] The deep peroneal nerve provides sensation to the webbing between the first and second digits and other than occasional variation, typically lies lateral to the anterior tibial artery on the anterior ankle.[51] The superficial peroneal nerve provides sensation to the dorsum of the foot and toes, except the first web space and typically travels anterior to the lateral malleolus at the ankle.[52] The sural nerve provides sensation to the posterolateral calf, ankle, and lateral foot and travels behind the lateral malleolus at the ankle.[53] The saphenous nerve provides sensation to the medial foot and ankle and may extend as far as the first digit. When it travels past the ankle it can be found in variable locations with variable branches, most of which travel over the medial malleoulus.[54] A complete ankle block requires 5 injections of local anesthetic; therefore, it is important to be cognizant of the local anesthetic used and maximum dosing to avoid local anesthetic toxicity. Because of variable anatomy and innervation of nerves in the foot and ankle, many ankle blocks require supplemental local anesthetic for pain control during procedures.[53,54]

Femoral nerve block The femoral nerve can be blocked in multiple locations along its course. The femoral nerve arises from the lumbar plexus and most often terminates at about the medial malleolus of the ankle as its terminal sensory branch, the saphenous nerve. Traditionally, the saphenous nerve was blocked with a below-the-knee field block but this technique had a poor success rate. Kent and colleagues[55] showed that using ultrasound significantly improved block success rates. One of the most common locations to block the saphenous nerve under ultrasound is in the adductor canal. Located in the middle third of the thigh, the adductor canal contains the saphenous nerve. The canal begins proximally at the apex of the femoral triangle and continues distally to the adductor hiatus.[56] Blocking the saphenous nerve in the adductor canal provides pain relief to the anterior inferior knee distal to the medial ankle.[57] It is useful for providing pain relief while sparing motor function of the quadriceps muscles.[56] In addition to the analgesia provided by the saphenous nerve block, blocking the femoral nerve at the inguinal crease provides analgesia to the anterior thigh and knee but decreases motor function of the quadriceps muscle.

Bauer and colleagues[58] revealed that decreasing the dose of local anesthetic for a femoral catheter can decrease quadriceps weakness, but the decreased weakness comes at the expense of adequate pain control. At the inguinal crease, the femoral nerve is located lateral to the femoral artery. The femoral artery is located near the femoral nerve for much of its course; therefore, care should be taken to avoid intravascular injection. As stated previously, the femoral nerve block at the inguinal crease will cause weakness of the quadriceps muscle and as such, can increase patient fall risk after regional anesthesia of the femoral nerve.[59]

Sciatic nerve block The sciatic nerve can be blocked at several locations along its course (**Fig. 2**). It arises from the sacral plexus, and its branches travel down the leg to provide sensory innervation to the posterior thigh and most of the lower leg and foot.[60] Good locations to block the sciatic nerve are at the bifurcation of the tibial and common peroneal nerves near the popliteal fossa, infragluteal, and gluteal. Blocking the sciatic nerve at the popliteal fossa is useful for surgery or pain control on the lower leg and foot. Performing the block after the bifurcation of the tibial nerve and common peroneal nerve may decrease the time required for onset of analgesia.[61] Blocking the sciatic nerve at the infragluteal location helps with pain control above the knee on the posterior thigh. The gluteal approach also anesthetizes the posterior thigh and provides a good location to place a nerve catheter, as it is not subject to as much motion as the infragluteal approach to the nerve.

Although the sciatic nerve has been blocked with landmarks and nerve stimulation for several decades, ultrasound offers improved block success, fewer needle redirections, decreased time to perform, and less procedural pain.[62] The sciatic nerve is a large nerve; therefore, adequate time must pass from local anesthetic injection before onset of analgesia, which can take upward of 30 minutes after performance of the block.[63] Given the large doses of local anesthetic that are sometimes used for regional anesthesia of the sciatic nerve, the proceduralist should be cognizant of the toxic dose

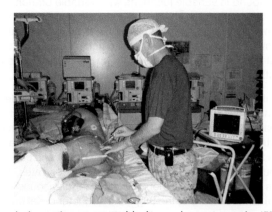

Fig. 2. Stimulator sciatic continuous nerve block on a lower extremity IED injury patient in Afghanistan. IED, improvised explosive device.

of the local anesthetic chosen for the procedure especially when combining the sciatic nerve block with femoral nerve regional anesthesia techniques. Efforts should be made to use the lowest effective dose of local anesthetic.[64] Jeong and colleagues[65] found that the effective dose of 0.5% ropivacaine for ultrasound-guided popliteal sciatic nerve blocks in 95% of patients undergoing foot and ankle surgery was 16 mL.

Neuraxial

Epidurals Epidurals are useful for pain control in trauma patients and can be used for lower extremity, abdominal, and thoracic injuries resulting from trauma. Transversus abdominus plane blocks may also be used for abdominal injuries or surgery (**Fig. 3**). Lumbar epidurals are frequently used in trauma patients with bilateral lower extremity injuries and can provide good analgesia for patients with extensive injuries that may require multiple surgical procedures. Patients receiving epidurals for major abdominal surgery have been found to have lower pain scores postsurgery and lower rates of respiratory failure.[66] Rib fractures are present in up to 10% of trauma patients admitted to trauma centers in the United States.[67] Controlling the pain from rib fractures is vitally important in trauma patients. Interestingly, Jensen and colleagues[68] found that despite having greater injury severity, thoracic epidural anesthesia predicted a 97% reduction in mortality for patients with thoracic epidural anesthesia and rib fractures versus those patients without epidurals. Not all studies of thoracic epidurals in rib fractures have found similar results; therefore, although thoracic epidurals may be useful in trauma patients, they are just one possible approach to the multimodal approach to pain control in these patients.[69] When epidural supplies are unavailable, paravertebral blocks (**Fig. 4**) can be useful for pain associated with thoracic and abdominal injuries and have been found to provide similar benefits in patients with rib fractures.[70]

Regional anesthesia and multimodal pain control

It is important to remember that regional anesthesia is only part of the multimodal plan for pain control in trauma patients. Given the severe pain frequently experienced by trauma patients, it is important to use all modalities of pain control. Historically, some of the oldest and most frequently used medications for pain relief in trauma patients have been opioids. Although opioids have a place in pain control for trauma patients, physicians have realized the importance of decreasing their use due to their side effects.[71] As a result, both nonopioid pain medications and acupuncture have

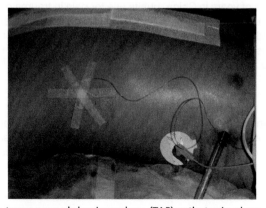

Fig. 3. Continuous transversus abdominus plane (TAP) catheter in place.

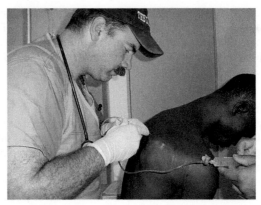

Fig. 4. Medical mission to Burkina Faso, Africa, providing paravertebral blocks for a scapular tumor.

been integrated into the care of trauma patients. One frequently used nonopioid medication is acetaminophen. In postsurgical patients, oral acetaminophen was shown to decrease opioid consumption on postsurgical day 1 by 22.6%.[72]

Alpha 2 agonists also have opioid sparing effects and are used for sedation in trauma patients. In a meta-analysis conducted by Blaudszun and colleagues,[73] clonidine decreased 24-hour postoperative morphine equivalent consumption by 4.1 mg, and dexmedetomidine deceased consumption by 14.5 mg. Ketamine is another opioid sparing medication that is used for trauma patients, especially in field environments. Ketamine is used for induction of anesthesia, pain relief, general anesthesia, and procedural sedation. Given ketamine's versatility, it is used in the care of injured patients in military and civilian prehospital settings.[74,75] Even in low doses, ketamine decreases opioid consumption when used as part of a multimodal approach to surgical pain.[76] Ketamine may also improve the symptoms of treatment resistant depression and posttraumatic stress disorder.[77] For all these reasons, ketamine should always be considered when creating a multimodal pain plan for trauma patients.

Although all medications to treat pain have their individual side effects, using a multimodal approach will help avoid the side effects of any one medication. A unique, nonpharmacologic therapy for pain management is acupuncture. Acupuncture has been used for thousands of years in China, but its use for pain in trauma patients in western medicine is relatively new.[8] It has been used for posttraumatic stress disorder, phantom limb pain, and neuropathy. It is attractive for use in field environments due to its portability, low cost, and minimal training to perform.[8] Acupuncture may provide pain relief while having no impact on a patient's ability to return to duty.[78]

SUMMARY

In the field, anesthesiologists can have an important role in relieving pain and facilitating surgical procedures. Regional anesthesia techniques are ideal in these situations, as they allow patients to maintain their cognitive and physical abilities, which can be crucial in times of disaster. If anesthesiologists adequately anticipate the patients and injuries that they will encounter, exploit the advantages of regional anesthesia, and mitigate the risks, they are an invaluable asset to medical care in the field for trauma victims.

CLINICS CARE POINTS

- Regional anesthesia can facilitate pain relief and surgical procedures while preserving a patient's mental and physical abilities.
- Every effort should be made to use standard ASA monitors in the field, but lack of these monitors should not deter use of regional anesthesia if the clinical situation warrants its use.
- Emergency airway equipment, cardiovascular medications, and lipid emulsion should be available when performing regional anesthesia in the field.
- Ultrasonography has improved the safety and success of regional anesthesia and should be used when available and indicated.
- Despite the dirty conditions frequently encountered in field environments, continuous peripheral nerve catheters are safe with proper aseptic technique.
- Continuous peripheral nerve block catheters and regional anesthesia decrease pain during transport of trauma patients.
- Regional anesthesia techniques decrease opioid consumption and their associated side effects.
- If performing continuous nerve block catheters and regional anesthesia in field environments, an acute pain management system should be in place to follow the patient from point of injury to definitive care.
- Regional anesthesia is only one portion of a multimodal approach to pain management in trauma patients.

REFERENCES

1. Botchey IM, Hung YW, Bachani AM, et al. Understanding patterns of injury in Kenya: analysis of a trauma registry data from a National Referral Hospital. Surgery 2017;162(6S):S54–62.
2. Heim C, Bosisio F, Roth A, et al. Is trauma in Switzerland any different? epidemiology and patterns of injury in major trauma - a 5-year review from a Swiss trauma centre. Swiss Med Wkly 2014;144:w13958.
3. Committee on Anesthesia Care Team. Guidelines, statements, clinical resources. American Society of Anesthesiologists. ASA Statement on Regional Anesthesia Web site. 2017. Available at: https://www.asahq.org/standards-and-guidelines/statement-on-regional-anesthesia. Accessed October 23, 2020.
4. Buckenmaier CC, McKnight GM, Winkley JV, et al. Continuous peripheral nerve block for battlefield anesthesia and evacuation. Reg Anesth Pain Med 2005;30: 202–5.
5. Scott DM. Regional anesthesia and analgesia on the front line. Anaesth Intensive Care 2009;37:1008–11.
6. Kent ML, Buckenmaier CC. Battlefield regional anesthesia: evolution and future concepts. Tech Reg Anesth Pain Manag 2012;16(4):184–9.
7. Buckenmaier CC, Lee EH, Shields CH, et al. Regional anesthesia in austere environments. Reg Anesth Pain Med 2003;28(4):321.
8. Buckenmaier CC, Bleckner LL, Sracic MK. Military advanced regional anesthesia and analgesia handbook. In: Lenhart MK, editor. Washington, DC: Office of the Surgeon General at TMM Publications; 2008. p. 25–79. Available at: http://www.dvcipm.org/clinical-resources/dvcipm-maraa-book-project/. Accessed October 23, 2020.

9. Buckenmaier CC, Mahoney PF, Anton T, et al. Impact of an acute pain service on pain outcomes with combat injured soldiers at Camp Bastion, Afghanistan. Pain Med 2012;13:919–26.

10. Carness JM, Wilson MA, Lenart MJ, et al. Experiences with regional anesthesia for analgesia during prolonged aeromedical evacuation. Aerosp Med Hum Perform 2017;88(8):768–72.

11. Ayling OG, Montbriand J, Jiang J, et al. Continuous regional anaesthesia provides effective pain management and reduces opioid requirement following major lower limb amputation. Eur J Vasc Endovasc Surg 2014;48(5):559–64.

12. Buckenmaier CC, Rupprecht C, McKnight G, et al. Pain following battlefield injury and evacuation: a survey of 110 casualties from the wars in Iraq and Afghanistan. Pain Med 2009;10(8):1487–96.

13. De Cassai A, Bonanno C, Sandei L, et al. PECS II block is associated with lower incidence of chronic pain after breast surgery. Korean J Pain 2019;32(4):286–91.

14. Jenson MG, Sorensen RF. Early use of regional and local anesthesia in a combat environment may prevent the development of complex regional pain syndrome in wounded combatants. Mil Med 2006;171(396):396–8.

15. Mathais Q, Montcriol A, Cotte J, et al. Anesthesia during deployment of a military forward surgical unit in low income countries: a register study of 1547 anesthesia cases. PLoS One 2019;14(10):e0223497.

16. Bleckner LL, Bina S, Kwon KH, et al. Serum ropivicaine concentrations and systemic local anesthetic toxicity in trauma patients receiving long-term continuous peripheral nerve block catheters. Anesthesia and Analgesia 2010;110(2):630–4.

17. Stojadinovic A, Auton A, Peoples GE, et al. Responding to challenges in modern combat casualty care innovative use of advanced regional anesthesia. Pain Med 2006;7:330–8.

18. Hebl JR. The importance and implications of aseptic techniques during regional anesthesia. Reg Anesth Pain Med 2006;31:311–23.

19. Bomberg H, Bayer I, Wagenpfeil S, et al. Prolonged catheter use and infection in regional anesthesia: a retrospective registry analysis. Anesthesiology 2018; 128(4):764–73.

20. Lai TT, Jager L, Jones BL, et al. Continuous peripheral nerve block catheter infections in combat related injuries a case report of five soldiers from OEF and OIF. Pain Med 2011;12:1676–81.

21. Neuburger M, Buttner J, Blumenthal S, et al. Inflammation and infection complications of 2285 perineural catheters: a prospective study. Acta Anaesthesiol Scand 2007;51(1):108–14.

22. Barrington MJ, Kluger R. Ultrasound guidance reduces the risk of local anesthetic systemic toxicity following peripheral nerve blockade. Reg Anesth Pain Med 2013;38(4):289–99.

23. Bomberg H, Wetjen L, Wagenpfeil S, et al. Risks and benefits of ultrasound, nerve stimulation and their combination for guiding peripheral nerve blocks: a retrospective registry analysis. Anesthesia and Analgesia 2018;127(4):1035–43.

24. Gelfand HJ, Ouanes JP, Lesley MR, et al. Analgesic efficacy of ultrasound-guided regional anesthesia: a meta-analysis. J Clin Anesth 2011;23(2):90–6.

25. Rozanski TA, Edmondson JM, Jones SB. Ultrasonography in a forward-deployed military hospital. Mil Med 2005;170:99–102.

26. Tsui B. Ultrasound guidance and nerve stimulation implications for the future practice of regional anesthesia. Can J Anaesth 2007;54:165–70.

27. Gray AT. Atlas of ultrasound guided regional anesthesia. Philadelphia: Meloni D; 2019.

28. Okur OM, Sener A, Kavakli HS, et al. Two injection digital block versus single sub-cutaneous palmar injection block for finger lacerations. Eur J Trauma Emerg Surg 2017;43(6):863–8.

29. Choi S, Cho YS, Kang B, et al. The difference of subcutaneous digital nerve block method efficacy according to injection location. Am J Emerg Med 2020; 38(1):95–8.

30. Sonohata M, Nagamine S, Maeda K, et al. Subcutaneous single injection digital block with epinephrine. Anesthesiol Res Pract 2012;2012:487650.

31. Calder K, Chung B, O'Brien C, et al. Bupivacaine digital blocks: how long is the pain relief and temperature elevation? Plast Reconstr Surg 2013;131(5): 1098–104.

32. Leversedge FJ, Moore TJ, Peterson BC, et al. Compartment syndrome of the upper extremity. J Hand Surg Am 2011;36(3):544–59 [quiz: 560].

33. Warman E, Lin J. Ultrasound-guided ulnar nerve block and radiolucent foreign body retrieval from the hand. Vis J Emerg Med 2019;16:1–2.

34. Sulaiman S, Soames R, Lamb C. Ulnar nerve cutaneous distribution in the palm: application to surgery of the hand. Clin Anat 2015;28(8):1022–8.

35. Unluer EE, Karagoz A, Unluer S, et al. Ultrasound-guided ulnar nerve block for boxer fractures. Am J Emerg Med 2016;34(8):1726–7.

36. Leis AA, Wells KJ. Radial nerve cutaneous innervation to the ulnar dorsum of the hand. Clin Neurophysiol 2008;119(3):662–6.

37. Frenkel O, Herring AA, Fischer J, et al. Supracondylar radial nerve block for treatment of distal radius fractures in the emergency department. J Emerg Med 2011; 41(4):386–8.

38. Ko JW, Mirarchi AJ. Late reconstruction of median nerve palsy. Orthop Clin North Am 2012;43(4):449–57.

39. Kokkalis ZT, Mavrogenis AF, Saranteas T, et al. Ultrasound-guided anterior axilla musculocutaneous nerve block. Radiol Med 2014;119(2):135–41.

40. Stone MB, Wang R, Price DD. Ultrasound-guided supraclavicular brachial plexus nerve block vs procedural sedation for the treatment of upper extremity emergencies. Am J Emerg Med 2008;26(6):706–10.

41. Gauss A, Tugtekin I, Georgieff M, et al. Incidence of clinically symptomatic pneumothorax in ultrasound-guided infraclavicular and supraclavicular brachial plexus block. Anaesthesia 2014;69(4):327–36.

42. Pham-Dang C, Gunst JP, Gouin F, et al. A novel supraclavicular approach to brachial plexus block. Anesth Analg 1997;85:111–6.

43. Blaivas M, Lyon M. Ultrasound-guided interscalene block for shoulder dislocation reduction in the ED. Am J Emerg Med 2006;24(3):293–6.

44. Buttner B, Mansur A, Kalmbach M, et al. Prehospital ultrasound-guided nerve blocks improve reduction-feasibility of dislocated extremity injuries compared to systemic analgesia. A randomized controlled trial. PLoS One 2018;13(7): e0199776.

45. Urmey WF, Talts KH, Sharrock NE. One hundred percent incidence of hemidiaphragmatic paresis associated with interscalene brachial plexus anesthesia as diagnosed by ultrasonography. Anesth Analg 1991;72:498–503.

46. Lee JH, Cho SH, Kim SH, et al. Ropivacaine for ultrasound-guided interscalene block: 5 mL provides similar analgesia but less phrenic nerve paralysis than 10 mL. Can J Anaesth 2011;58(11):1001–6.

47. Passannante AN. Spinal anesthesia and permanent neurologic deficit after interscalene block. Anesth Analg 1996;82:873–4.

48. Lopez AM, Sala-Blanch X, Magaldi M, et al. Ultrasound-guided ankle block for forefoot surgery: the contribution of the saphenous nerve. Reg Anesth Pain Med 2012;37(5):554–7.

49. Chin KJ, Wong NW, Macfarlane AJ, et al. Ultrasound-guided versus anatomic landmark-guided ankle blocks: a 6-year retrospective review. Reg Anesth Pain Med 2011;36(6):611–8.

50. Wassef MR. Posterior tibial nerve block A new approach using the bony landmarks fo the sustenaculum tali. Anaesthesia 1991;46(10):841.

51. Antonakakis JG, Scalzo DC, Jorgenson AS, et al. Ultrasound does not improve the success rate of a deep peroneal nerve block at the ankle. Reg Anesth Pain Med 2010;35(2):217–21.

52. Tzika M, Paraskevas G, Natsis KN. Entrapment of the superficial peroneal nerve. J Am Podiatr Med Assoc 2015;105:150–9.

53. Jeon SK, Paik DJ, Hwang YI. Variations in sural nerve formation pattern and distribution on the dorsum of the foot. Clin Anat 2017;30(4):525–32.

54. Marsland D, Dray A, Little NJ, et al. The saphenous nerve in foot and ankle surgery: its variable anatomy and relevance. Foot Ankle Surg 2013;19(2):76–9.

55. Kent ML, Hackworth RJ, Riffenburgh RH, et al. A comparison of ultrasound-guided and landmark-based approaches to saphenous nerve blockade: a prospective, controlled, blinded, crossover trial. Anesth Analg 2013;117(1):265–70.

56. Seo SS, Kim OG, Seo JH, et al. Comparison of the effect of continuous femoral nerve block and adductor canal block after primary total knee arthroplasty. Clin Orthop Surg 2017;9(3):303–9.

57. Mistry D, O'Meeghan C. Fate of the infrapatellar branch of the saphenous nerve post total knee arthroplasty. ANZ J Surg 2005;75(9):822–4.

58. Bauer M, Wang L, Onibonoje OK, et al. Continuous femoral nerve blocks decreasing local anesthetic concentration to minimize quadriceps femoris weakness. Anesthesiology 2012;V(3):665–72.

59. Ranawat A. Preoperative femoral nerve block did not reduce oral opioid consumption at 24 hours and increased risk of noninjurious falls after hip arthroscopy. J Bone Joint Surg Am 2016;98(16):1407.

60. Distad BJ, Weiss MD. Clinical and electrodiagnostic features of sciatic neuropathies. Phys Med Rehabil Clin N Am 2013;24(1):107–20.

61. Faiz SHR, Imani F, Rahimzadeh P, et al. Which ultrasound-guided sciatic nerve block strategy works faster? Prebifurcation or separate tibial-peroneal nerve block? A randomized clinical trial. Anesth Pain Med 2017;7(4):e57804.

62. Danelli G, Fanelli A, Ghisi D, et al. Ultrasound vs nerve stimulation multiple injection technique for posterior popliteal sciatic nerve block. Anaesthesia 2009;64(6):638–42.

63. Taboada M, Alvarez J, Cortes J, et al. The effects of three different approaches on the onset time of sciatic nerve blocks with 0.75% ropivacaine. Anesth Analg 2004;98(1):242–7.

64. Bang SU, Kim DJ, Bae JH, et al. Minimum effective local anesthetic volume for surgical anesthesia by subparaneural, ultrasound-guided popliteal sciatic nerve block: a prospective dose-finding study. Medicine (Baltimore) 2016;95(34):e4652.

65. Jeong JS, Shim JC, Jeong MA, et al. Minimum effective anaesthetic volume of 0.5% ropivacaine for ultrasound-guided popliteal sciatic nerve block in patients undergoing foot and ankle surgery: determination of ED50 and ED95. Anaesth Intensive Care 2015;43:92–7.

66. Rigg JRA, Jamrozik K, Myles PS, et al. Epidural anaesthesia and analgesia and outcome of major surgery: a randomised trial. Lancet 2002;359(9314):1276–82.
67. Ziegler DW, Agarwal NN. The morbidity and mortality of rib fractures. J Trauma 1994;37:975–9.
68. Jensen CD, Stark JT, Jacobson LL, et al. Improved outcomes associated with the liberal use of thoracic epidural analgesia in patients with rib fractures. Pain Med 2017;18(9):1787–94.
69. Galvagno SM, Smith CE, Varon AJ, et al. Pain management for blunt thoracic trauma: a joint practice management guideline from the Eastern Association for the Surgery of Trauma and Trauma Anesthesiology Society. J Trauma Acute Care Surg 2016;81(5):936–51.
70. Malekpour M, Hashmi A, Dove J, et al. Analgesic choice in management of rib fractures: paravertebral block or epidural analgesia? Anesth Analg 2017; 124(6):1906–11.
71. Smith JE, Russell RR, Mahoney PF, et al. What is the ideal pre-hospital analgesic a questionaire study. J R Army Med Corps 2009;155:42–67.
72. Wasserman I, Poeran J, Zubizarreta N, et al. Impact of intravenous acetaminophen on perioperative opioid utilization and outcomes in open colectomies: a claims database analysis. Anesthesiology 2018;129(1):77–88.
73. Blaudszun G, Lysakowski C, Nadia Elia, et al. Effect of perioperative systemic alpha 2 agonists on postoperative morphine consumption and pain intensity. Pain Med 2012;116(6):1312–22.
74. Bredmose PP, Lockey DJ, Grier G, et al. Pre-hospital use of ketamine for analgesia and procedural sedation. Emerg Med J 2009;26(1):62–4.
75. Moy R, Wright C. Ketamine for military prehospital analgesia and sedation in combat casualties. J R Army Med Corps 2018;164(6):436–7.
76. Gharaei B, Jafari A, Aghamohammadi H, et al. Opioid-sparing effect of preemptive bolus low-dose ketamine for moderate sedation in opioid abusers undergoing extracorporeal shock wave lithotripsy: a randomized clinical trial. Anesth Analg 2013;116(1):75–80.
77. Hartberg J, Garrett-Walcott S, De Gioannis A. Impact of oral ketamine augmentation on hospital admissions in treatment-resistant depression and PTSD: a retrospective study. Psychopharmacology (Berl) 2018;235(2):393–8.
78. Niemtzow RC. Battlefield acupuncture. New Rochelle (NY): Medical Acupuncture; 2007. p. 1–12.

Resident Education and Redeployment During a Disaster

Vanessa Mazandi, MD[a],*, Emily Gordon, MD, MSEd[b]

KEYWORDS

- Resident education • Anesthesia residency • COVID-19 • Housestaff
- Resident staffing model

KEY POINTS

- Redefining roles for anesthesia residents in a pandemic.
- Preparing residents to take on new roles during a time of limited health care resources.
- Balancing clinical service and education during a time of limited health care resources.
- Providing emotional support for residents during a health care crisis.

INTRODUCTION

In the United States, there are more than 140,000 physician residents training in more than 20 specialties.[1] Many are in US cities with more than 8000 people per square mile; locations with population densities that make them more susceptible to spread of a pathogen via droplet or airborne methods. When a virulent microorganism with high communicability hits regions of high population density, there exists the potential for an epidemic, which can pose a threat to the stability of the health system in these communities. As the spread of the novel severe acute respiratory syndrome coronavirus 2 (SARS-CoV-2; Coronavirus Disease 2019 [COVID-19]) has demonstrated, our global economy provides the runway, so to speak, for an epidemic to enter the category of pandemic, with the ability to disrupt health care systems worldwide.

In the US health care system, resident physicians make up more than 10% of the physician work force,[2] a proportion that grows larger if you compare resident physicians with inpatient-based attending physicians. Furthermore, as larger hospitals can accommodate a higher number of trainees in residency programs, most resident physicians practice at tertiary medical centers that assume care for the sickest, most

[a] Department of Anesthesiology and Critical Care, Children's Hospital of Philadelphia, 3401 Civic Center Boulevard, Philadelphia, PA 19104, USA; [b] Department of Anesthesiology and Critical Care, Hospital of the University of Pennsylvania, 3400 Spruce Street, Philadelphia, PA 19104, USA
* Corresponding author.
E-mail address: mazandiv@email.chop.edu

Anesthesiology Clin 39 (2021) 353–361
https://doi.org/10.1016/j.anclin.2021.02.007
1932-2275/21/© 2021 Elsevier Inc. All rights reserved.
anesthesiology.theclinics.com

complex patients; patients who are most vulnerable in a pandemic. Given their large footprint within the US health care system, the specialty-specific skill sets, ability to care for patients in novel environments, and educational requirements of residents are all factors that must be considered when determining how best to use these physicians-in-training to ensure outstanding patient care both in the short-term scope of a pandemic surge, and in the future as trainees assume the role of attending physicians.

At the same time, although it is true that a career in medicine entails lifelong learning, resident physicians have unique needs among learners in that they are building the necessary foundations of the educational base that will serve them for their careers. Not only is it important that their skillsets be redeployed in useful ways during a crisis that stresses the health care system, but it is equally as critical that their overall educational goals are met. COVID-19 created additional stress for resident education, forcing creative solutions to continue resident education during a time when the tug-of-war between clinical duties and didactics intensified. A highly communicable disease, COVID-19 required renewed commitment to ensure time for didactic learning, while also finding ways to keep it effective in a remote learning environment. The lessons learned during the COVID-19 outbreak in the spring of 2020 can be applied to any disaster that challenges the US health system.

Among resident physicians, those in anesthesia face unique challenges in a pandemic given their skillset. Anesthesia residents are well-suited to care for patients in a critical care environment as front-line ordering clinicians both from a medical management standpoint, and due to familiarity with ordering processes given their role as residents, and relatively recent roles as interns and medical students, within a large hospital structure. In addition, anesthesiology requires mastery of procedural skills, which can be more difficult to attain when elective surgical cases are canceled to enable better resource utilization within the hospital during a pandemic. Anesthesia residents serve as a fluid work force that can quickly adapt to a critical care environment. The additional benefit of staffing anesthesia residents in the intensive care unit (ICU) is the educational value for the trainees in the setting of fewer operating room (OR) cases. As will be discussed further, clinical/"bedside" learning is challenging during a pandemic that requires socially distanced virtual learning; rotating through the ICU provides an opportunity for anesthesia residents to use and improve on their procedural and critical thinking skills.

DISCUSSION: REDEPLOYMENT OF RESIDENTS

Anesthesia residents are uniquely suited to redeployment during a pandemic that requires specialists in critical care. The more than 6700 anesthesia residents[1] in the United States provide valuable staffing during times when the resources of the health care system are challenged. Not only do anesthesia residents have high exposure to equipment and procedures used to care for critically ill patients (including ventilators, advanced airways, and advanced monitoring devices, as well as arterial and central line placement) but they have more recent exposure to different areas of the hospital, including specific ICU rotations, and potentially even different electronic medical record systems given their proximity to medical school rotations. As such, they are distinctively qualified to serve as front-line care providers in the ICU as they are both familiar with the ICU environment, and have recent exposure to a variety of medical environments and electronic medical records.

In fact, because anesthesia residents possess a skillset that makes them adaptable to working in non-OR locations caring for critically ill patients, their absence from other rotations must be weighed in the setting of limited resources. For example, during a pandemic-driven surge in hospital admissions, it may be more appropriate to have a junior medicine resident help with the duties of the pain service or perioperative clinic so that anesthesia residents can be prioritized for staffing needs in the ICU. In addition, senior anesthesia residents can be relied on to serve, alongside advanced practice practitioners (APPs), as supervisors within the front-line ordering clinician hierarchy given the exposure to ICU monitoring and life-sustaining interventions that are encountered in daily OR assignments. This ability for supervision and service as educators becomes especially important when hospitals are forced to shift to a pandemic/mass casualty event model of staffing, where residents are pulled from normal assignments to cover areas of the hospital with which they may have less familiarity.

During the initial COVID-19 outbreak in the spring of 2020, elective surgical cases were canceled, leaving an abundance of surgical residents with decreased clinical duties, available to fill other roles in the hospital (**Figs. 1** and **2**). Even on nonsurgical floors, the spring of 2020 COVID-19 experience demonstrated how quickly all hospital services can have a decrease in other types of admissions during a pandemic, increasing the number of trainees available to work in an ICU setting.[3–5] In addition, as was seen in New York City and London during the spring of 2020 COVID-19 outbreak, pediatric ICUs can provide valuable beds during a surge in illness that affects adults more severely than children.[6] In settings in which adult patients were cared for in a pediatric setting, front-line ordering clinicians included general pediatrics residents. Although surge spaces, whether in a pediatric ICU, OR, or medical or surgical floor, provide critical bed capacity, it is important that the providers caring for patients are equipped to care for these, at times, unfamiliar patient populations in an equitable fashion. This is just as important at the attending physician and nursing levels as it is for the front-line ordering clinicians. Although redistribution of health care resources can create increased staffing in a pandemic surge model, residents and APPs with limited critical care experience will benefit from being on teams with anesthesia colleagues as well as ICU-trained APPs.

Another key component to "uptraining" faculty, trainees, and other providers during the pandemic was Penn's creation of a front-facing, public Web site with curriculums developed based on the provider's prior knowledge and area of redeployment.[7] During a time when ICU fellows and attending physicians may be following as many as 50 patients at a time, anesthesia residents and APPs, as both colleagues and

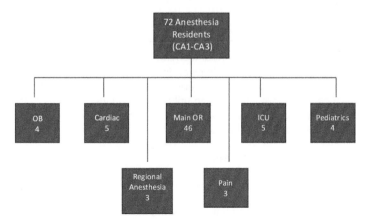

Fig. 1. Pre-COVID anesthesia resident staffing model.

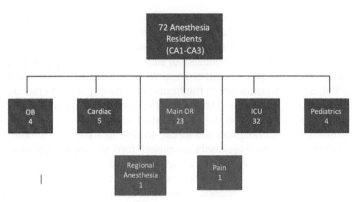

Fig. 2. COVID anesthesia resident staffing model.

supervisors, can provide education to those less familiar in critical care environments and help to ensure quality metrics are being met for all patients.

Efficacy within this ICU role is best met with preparation. The Department of Anesthesiology and Critical Care at the Hospital of the University of Pennsylvania (HUP) groomed the department's residents for their roles in the ICU by rotating small groups of residents for a brief time of 2 to 5 days through the ICUs. This served to both familiarize them with various ICU environments (including ICUs where they had not previously rotated), and develop camaraderie with the APPs and nurses. The time before a potential surge was the most valuable window in which to do this integration, as it ensured not only good care of patients with COVID-19, but also patients having urgent surgeries that required detailed, attentive care from practitioners familiar with their postoperative courses and possible complications.

As the surge intensified 100 miles north of Philadelphia, patients from New York and New Jersey were brought to University of Pennsylvania Health System hospitals, increasing the number of patients with COVID-19 and likewise the need for isolated units to care for the infected patients. Newer surge spaces were created, including a 36-bed negative-pressure unit in the postoperative care unit [PACU] of the HUP. Residents, APPs, and faculty who would work in this unit were notified ahead of time and participated in simulations within the unit before its opening. Although the PACU-turned-ICU was fortunately not needed in the spring of 2020 COVID-19 outbreak, the simulations were beneficial to establish the roles of anesthesia residents within this unit, and develop familiarity with the nurses and APPs who would work alongside them. In addition, an opportunity was leveraged for resident education with inclusion of the residents in virtual learning within the Division of Critical Care. There were also in-person demonstrations of different ventilators presented by critical care fellows, faculty, and respiratory therapists. During a time when OR cases were drastically reduced, resident learning and utilization continued in ways that prepared anesthesia trainees to be both board-certified anesthesiologists and front-line ordering clinicians in the event of a pandemic.

RESIDENT EDUCATION IN A PANDEMIC

The necessary cancellation of elective surgeries interrupted a critical component of clinical learning for anesthesia residents. At the same time, social distancing reduced the ability for didactic learning to continue in-person. The second problem was more easily addressed than the first.

Had COVID-19 presented itself 20 years ago, the ramifications on resident education could have been more damaging. However, within the anesthesia residency program at HUP, all the residents had access to the Internet and computers within their homes, making it possible to convert didactics to an online forum using the platforms BlueJeans and Zoom. Although the virtual learning environment cannot replace in-person learning, fortunately case conferences, board question reviews, and mock oral boards were able to continue with use of the chat function, selective muting of participants, and screen share for PowerPoint presentations.

The lack of in-person didactics combined with a less rigorous OR schedule allowed time to create a comprehensive resident educational Web site with video tutorials and didactics that will continue to be a resource, regardless of social distancing measures. A department-specific intranet that is updated in a timely fashion also can serve as a communication platform. The intranet can be a place to give updates, as well as post videos to demonstrate for all members of the department the skills necessary in the pandemic, such as proper donning and doffing of personal protective equipment, when to wear an N-95 mask and eye protection during intubations, and how to use filters with Ambu bags and the anesthesia machine when delivering care to infected patients. The residency leadership at HUP took advantage of a change in normal routines to enhance the available education resources. Building this type of infrastructure adds value to resident education in "normal times"; it becomes invaluable within the context of a pandemic. Real-time feedback was provided with regard to the new resident virtual curriculum in the form of weekly town halls with residency leadership.

Clinical learning is one of the most important aspects of resident education, especially for anesthesia. Although the ICU environment is a natural place for residents to expand their knowledge and skills in the use of vasoactive medications, sedatives, resuscitation pathophysiology, and vascular access, certain aspects of clinical knowledge are difficult to replicate during a pandemic. Regional anesthesia is one such specialty that requires clinical exposure and was adversely affected during the pandemic. Most blocks performed during a regional anesthesia rotation are done for elective orthopedic surgeries, which are often the first types of cases to be canceled when a crisis hits the health care system. Even with flexibility allowed by the American College of Graduate Medical Education (ACGME) for minimum number of blocks performed required to graduate from residency, acquiring proficiency in a time of limited elective cases is still a concern.

In times where resident presence is prioritized in other areas of the hospital, a more creative and personalized scheduling strategy is required. During a time when less regional anesthesia is done, it can be beneficial to have fewer residents on the rotation for less time; thus, cycling more residents through during, say, a 3-month stretch while allowing a single resident to handle the reduced volume of blocks during their rotation time. Prioritizing residents who have a strong interest in regional anesthesia, or who need more numbers of regional pain blocks, can also help to create an equitable system during a time of reduced learning opportunities. During the peak of COVID-19 cases in Philadelphia, the regional anesthesia rotation that normally has 2 residents, had only 1 assigned for usually a week at a time. When elective cases resumed, priority for the rotation was given to those who needed block numbers, and to those who had indicated a strong interest in regional anesthesia.

In addition to specialty rotations that are adversely impacted during a pandemic, foundational knowledge can be adversely affected. A mainstay of learning anesthesia is the introduction to the specialty through "one to ones." At HUP, clinical anesthesia-1 (CA-1) residents are assigned to an attending in a 1-to-1 ratio during the month of July during a rotation called "1:1s." In preparation for the springtime COVID-19 surge, there was concern that 1:1s may not be able to continue in traditional fashion if there was still cessation of elective cases during the summer. Fortunately, the HUP ORs were at nearly full capacity in July 2020, and 1:1s proceeded as planned. However, COVID-19 provided an opportunity to reflect on how 1:1s could occur during a health care crisis with reduced surgical volume. Our 1:1s primarily consist of OR time and so with fewer elective cases, it may have required that the intensive training occur over a period of 2 to 3 months rather than 1 month. To allow some autonomy as well as flexibility for resident staffing, a system of milestones could be used to allow some independent practice of residents (under attending medical direction) within this 2-month to 3-month timespan. For example, while a CA-1 having successfully completed 1:1s could be under the medical direction of an attending physician for a variety of cases, in a setting with reduced volume, the same CA-1 could be cleared to care for American Society of Anesthesiologists 1 and 2 patients in the outpatient surgery center under medical direction. This would allow for some autonomy and growth in the OR with the expectation that they would still have periods in which they shift back to the 1:1 model during this 2-month to 3-month training period to gain competency in a variety of cases. This benchmark-driven approach to completion of 1:1s would enable safe patient care to continue, while making the most of lower case volumes and allowing attending physicians to be more available to medically direct and work in the ICUs rather than having a full class of 1:1s to instruct at any one time.

During times of especially low OR case volume, it is possible that even with a rotation system with oscillation between 1:1 instruction and medically directed practice, there may not be enough OR cases to provide learning opportunities for all the new CA-1s at the same time. In this scenario, an alternative could be to have some of the new CA-1 residents work with senior anesthesia residents in the ICUs where they can be prioritized to place vascular access lines, intubate (when appropriate for COVID-19–negative patients or times when there is no increased risk of transmission with aerosol-generating procedures) and learn more about medications that are used with frequency in the ICU and OR. To ensure quality and some measure of standardization in the curriculum, senior residents in the ICU could have a list of skills and topics to cover with CA-1s, just as attending anesthesiologists currently have in the OR setting. During a time when there are not enough elective OR cases for all CA-1s to learn at the same time, although not ideal, increasing the time of 1:1s and pairing CA-1s with senior residents who have been pulled to the ICUs can mitigate the loss of learning that occurs for future critical workers in the health care system.

Although necessary deployment to the ICU in a pandemic can serve as an opportunity to expand the anesthesia skillset, there will still be compromise of resident learning when elective OR cases are canceled. Simulation is a valuable tool to improve learning and teamwork.[8,9] Using simulation to mimic normal OR settings for CA-1s with abbreviated 1:1s can accelerate learning in an environment with low OR volumes. In addition, the same principles can be applied for other CA-2 and CA-3 specialties that have lower volumes during a pandemic. Simulations that provide opportunities to troubleshoot a double-lumen endotracheal tube in a thoracic case, or manage a Type 2 protamine reaction in a cardiac case, will never replace learning in the setting of direct patient care. Nonetheless, simulation has a role to strengthen critical thinking skills and supplement clinical learning in the ICU while opportunities for clinical learning in the OR are decreased. Well-planned simulations can provide a productive use of the extra time afforded by a slower OR schedule.

Resident Mental Health in a Pandemic

COVID-19 brought the issue of physician burnout to the public consciousness. In the medical arena, if it was not already discussed, it became a more prominent topic.

COVID-19 served to intensify issues the medical field had with mental health and well-being.[10] Mental well-being in anesthesiology is especially significant because poor mental health can be a risk factor for drug abuse in a specialty where there is access to addictive medications. Anesthesiology residents are at particular risk of substance use/abuse, with an incidence of 1% to 2% per year.[11] Regardless of whether substance use is an endpoint, mental health of residents during particularly stressful times, such as a pandemic, must be addressed. At HUP, the chief residents held weekly town halls over a virtual platform with program leadership oftentimes joining for the last 10 to 15 minutes to answer questions from the residents that could not be addressed by the chiefs. In addition, fortuitously, at the beginning of the 2019 to 2020 academic year (AY), the chief residents had divided the residents into 3 groups of "families," 1 for each chief resident to oversee. These groups spanned class years and provided a platform for residents to get to know each other across classes outside of work, and have a chief with whom they could always feel comfortable going to with concerns. COVID-19 began to surge in the United States just as the 2019 to 2020 AY anesthesia chiefs at Penn were transitioning duties to the newly selected 2020 to 2021 AY chiefs. This transition allowed each chief family to have 2 chiefs at the helm (both incoming and outgoing), which allowed each of the 6 chiefs to have 13 to 14 residents to reach out to individually on a weekly basis. Thus, the town halls allowed for weekly updates to schedule changes and provided a forum for concerns to be aired to the group. The weekly individual check-ins allowed the chiefs to assess which residents had notable challenges, fears, and/or concerns associated with the pandemic and assess which residents could use additional support. Dividing the residents among the 6 chiefs also allowed for rapid dissemination of news as it came in. The chief families provided the template for a phone tree; rather than wait for the weekly departmental town halls, chiefs could directly contact their 13 to 14 residents to deliver salient updates.

In addition to personalized check-ins, the department ensured that everyone (residents and faculty) was aware of the mental health resources available to them through the hospital system. However, although having information about these resources was important, during the COVID-19 surge, many of these resources were overwhelmed and unable to provide timely care to residents in need. The personalized check-ins allowed for better identification of residents who were struggling and for those who were, our department chair worked quickly to provide access to mental health services outside of the traditional resources. In addition, faculty who were in quarantine due to clinical exposure, were quick to offer their services if residents or faculty needed someone to speak with confidentially about their personal and professional difficulties during the COVID-19 surge. This had the dual effect of not only helping the residents, but also the side-lined faculty, who felt powerless to help their colleagues while quarantined at home for 14 days. The department ombudsmen continued to provide a space for residents to bring concerns. Although discussing mental health remains a stigma in medicine, the Department of Anesthesiology and Critical Care at Penn continued a tradition of emphasizing its importance during the COVID-19 pandemic and provided multiple outlets, including one-on-one conversations, for residents to be heard.

SUMMARY

In summary, COVID-19 challenged the US health care system in a way that its predecessors (including SARS-CoV-1, Middle Eastern Respiratory Syndrome, and H1N1) had not. Not only did it strain the health care system and cause cancellation of elective surgeries to accommodate increased numbers of patients, but it also threatened the work force.

In our global economy, it is unlikely that COVID-19 is an outlier. Whether it be future outbreaks of COVID-19 or a novel pathogen, it is almost a certainty that the US health care system will face another challenge to its resources, and most likely it will require those in anesthesiology and critical care to be at the forefront of the response. With a rapidly spreading disease like COVID-19, it is difficult to stay abreast as new knowledge about the novel pathogen evolves. With COVID-19, rapid shifts in our collective understanding of the disease, including the transmission mechanism, underscored the importance of having plans ready for future surges of COVID19 or another pathogen. A silver lining of COVID-19 is it allowed residency programs and hospital systems to rethink resident roles and assignments in the setting of an event that causes major strain on the health care system. COVID-19 underlined the importance of regular communication and transparency from leadership, not only for mental health but also as safety mechanisms, such as patient isolation, testing, contact tracing, and critically, personal protective equipment recommendations changed. Early prevention of spread with quick transitions to remote education is key; early preparedness with reimagining and retraining residents to fill specific roles ahead of time is equally important.

It is critical that departments have plans in place for how to use and educate anesthesia residents during a stress equal to, or greater than, the magnitude of disruption caused by COVID-19. Anesthesia residents possess specific skills that allow them to be key parts of the teams caring for patients. For this reason, their continued education during a time of crisis is important because it will enable them to be part of the next wave of attending physicians and educators on which the health care system relies.

DISCLOSURE

The authors have nothing to disclose.

REFERENCES

1. Accreditation Council for Graduate Medical Education. Data resource book: academic year 2019-2020. Chicago: ACGME; 2020. p. 49.
2. Young A, Chaudhry HJ, Pei X, et al. FSMB census of licensed physicians in the United States, 2018. J Med Regul 2018;105(2):7–23.
3. Huynh K. Reduced hospital admissions for ACS – more collateral damage from COVID-19. Nat Rev Cardiol 2020;17(8):453.
4. Jeffery M, D'Onofrio G, Paek H, et al. Trends in emergency department visits and hospital admissions in health care systems in 5 states in the first months of the COVID-19 pandemic in the US. JAMA Intern Med 2020;180(10):1328–33.
5. Diegoli H, Magalhães PSC, Martins SCO, et al. Decrease in hospital admissions for transient ischemic attack, mild, and moderate stroke during the COVID-19 era. Stroke 2020;51(8):2315–21.
6. Remy KE, Verhoef PA, Malone JR, et al. Caring for critically ill adults with coronavirus disease 2019 in a PICU: recommendations by dual trained intensivists. Pediatr Crit Care Med 2020;21(7):607–19.
7. UPHS Covid-19 Learning Website. Available at: https://www.med.upenn.edu/uphscovid19education/.
8. Lorello GR, Cook DA, Johnson RL, et al. Simulation-based training in anaesthesiology: a systematic review and meta-analysis. Br J Anaesth 2019;112(2):231–45.

9. Kolawole H, Guttormsen AB, Hepner DL, et al. Use of simulation to improve management of perioperative anaphylaxis: a narrative review. Br J Anaesth 2019; 123(1):e104–9.

10. Stuijfzand S, Deforges C, Sandoz V, et al. Psychological impact of an epidemic/ pandemic on the mental health of healthcare professionals: a rapid review. BMC Public Health 2020;20(1):1230.

11. Fitzsimons MG, Baker K, Malhotra R, et al. Reducing the incidence of substance use disorders in anesthesiology residents: 13 years of comprehensive urine drug screening. Anesthesiology 2018;129(4):821–8.

Anesthetic Resource Limitations and Adaptations in Times of Shortage

Experiences from New York Presbyterian Hospital During COVID-19

David S. Wang, MD*, Jonathan Hastie, MD,
Gebhard Wagener, MD, Oliver Panzer, MD

KEYWORDS

• COVID-19 • Pandemic staffing • ORICU • New York Presbyterian

KEY POINTS

- The COVID-19 pandemic surge in March 2020 strained the New York Presbyterian-Columbia system.
- The Department of Anesthesiology continued to manage emergency surgical cases and obstetrics while expanding airway management and novel intensive care unit coverage throughout the system.
- Resource limitations were material, physical, and staffing.

INTRODUCTION

The first confirmed case of coronavirus disease 2019 (COVID-19) in New York City (NYC) occurred in March 2020. Because the virus had been spreading undetected in the community, confirmed cases then grew exponentially. Over the next 2 months, the NYC metropolitan area became the worldwide epicenter. At its peak in April, COVID-19 was responsible for more than 500 deaths per day in NYC. As of October 2020, there have been 241,403 confirmed cases and 19,211 confirmed deaths from COVID-19[1] (https://www1.nyc.gov/site/doh/covid/covid-19-data.page).

As cases surged, New York-Presbyterian Hospital (NYP) oriented most of its clinical departments around care of COVID-19 patients. The hospital faced significant resource limitations that required rapid adaptation. The Department of Anesthesiology was immersed in this effort, and stewardship of resources impacted its operations of

Department of Anesthesiology, Columbia University Irving Medical Center, 630 West 168th Street, New York, NY 10032, USA
* Corresponding author.
E-mail address: Dsw2144@cumc.columbia.edu

Anesthesiology Clin 39 (2021) 363–377
https://doi.org/10.1016/j.anclin.2021.03.003   **anesthesiology.theclinics.com**
1932-2275/21/© 2021 Elsevier Inc. All rights reserved.

perioperative care, airway and cardiac arrest team, and intensive care unit (ICU) management. These resources related to materials (eg, medications, personal protective equipment [PPE], and ventilators), space, and personnel.

These efforts were complicated by significant ambiguity: at the time, optimal management and therapies were far from clear, and little was known about the true risks and vector of transmission between patients and health care workers (HCW). Resource management was a balancing act between the current situation, in which safety of patients and staff was paramount, and the forthcoming surge in NYC, which would be of unknown duration and intensity. Even if specific resource limitations could be addressed acutely, contingencies had to be made if the disease surge reached an even higher peak or lasted months to years.

In this article, the authors discuss their experiences at NYP-Columbia University Irving Medical Center (NYP-Columbia) as they addressed these resource limitations during the initial surge from March through May 2020.

GOALS

The department of anesthesiology is one of the larger departments at NYP-Columbia. It includes approximately 115 full-time attending anesthesiologists, and 19 of them are subspecialty trained in critical care medicine. Among trainees were approximately 100 residents and 9 critical care medicine fellows. Under usual conditions, the department staffs the postanesthesia care unit (PACU) and 47 surgical ICU beds using a closed care model. Because airway management and critical care are paramount in an epidemic with predominantly respiratory symptoms, the department aimed to allocate personnel with diverse skillsets to provide care as broadly as possible.

In the initial phases of the pandemic during March, this meant simply keeping up with the large influx of patients with COVID-19 adult respiratory distress syndrome (ARDS) requiring intubation and weeks-long ICU stays, in addition to providing the standard level of care to non–COVID-19 patients (eg, labor and delivery). As the capacity of ICU beds and ventilators threatened to reach its maximum, we spearheaded the conversion of operating room (OR) space into a temporary operating room intensive care unit (ORICU) and provided most of the medical staffing.

As the number of critically ill hospitalized patients began to plateau, our focus shifted from sheer capacity to quality improvement, with the aim of ensuring the same level of care in ORICU as in traditional ICUs.

Throughout this process, we recognized that safety of our staff was complementary to our goals of providing high-quality care. We believed that the best care delivery required that staff members be healthy, rested, and engaged. By prioritizing both the physical and the mental safety of our HCWs, our goal was to combat attrition and ensure a healthy workforce particularly during the initial phase when the duration and extent of the COVID-19 surge in NYC were unclear.

APPLICATION
Operating Rooms

On March 14, elective surgical procedures were canceled in New York State, and so the case load was limited to emergency surgery[2] (https://columbiasurgery.org/news/regarding-covid-19). At NYP-Columbia, we scaled down our anesthesia sites to a total of 6 ORs, with one dedicated to COVID-19–positive patients or patients under investigation (PUIs) who needed surgical procedures. With the limited case volume, 6 ORs were sufficient throughout the surge. Preoperative and postoperative care was given in the preoperative area to minimize patient transport through parts of the hospital with

COVID-19 patients. With the cancellation of elective procedures, surgical case volume was reduced greater than 90%, and many of our perioperative services, such as the acute pain service, were deployed elsewhere, mostly in the ORICU. Our major adaptations are summarized in **Table 1**, with further discussion in the later paragraphs.

PPE was stored in various central locations, and the disbursement was staffed by an HCW to ensure equitable distribution. NYP-Columbia had adequate N95 masks for all HCWs, but masks designed to be single use were reused multiple times by a single HCW. Single-use masks reused multiple times was achieved by wearing a surgical mask over the N95. Some HCWs used the N95 for up to 2 weeks. For all COVID-19 patients or PUIs, standard contact/droplet/airborne isolation precautions were strictly followed in the OR: surgical mask with N95 mask underneath, bouffant cap, fluid shield, and isolation gowns and gloves were worn by all HCWs in the rooms. For non–COVID-19 patients, these precautions were technically not required; however, almost all HCWs continued to at least wear N95 masks with fluid shields, particularly because testing was limited in the very beginning of the pandemic.

In addition to PPE and dedicated COVID-19/PUI ORs, the Department of Anesthesiology took several additional precautions. For all operative cases in the COVID-19–designated room, the anesthesia cart was covered with plastic drapes to minimize contact spread and then fully moved out into the sterile core. All anticipated medications and equipment that were likely to be used were kept in the room and stored on the anesthesia machine, to be discarded at the end of the case. Emergency medications (eg, epinephrine and atropine) were kept in a separate sealed plastic bag; the entire contents of this bag would be discarded at the end of the case if the bag were opened. This limited accessibility had the benefit of providing an additional layer of security by preventing potentially contaminated gloves from reaching into the cart routinely.

Contamination of the anesthesia machines with severe acute respiratory syndrome coronavirus 2 (SARS-CoV-2) was a major concern. At NYP-Columbia, we use King Systems anesthesia circuits, which have built-in bacterial/viral filters on both the

---

Table 1
Perioperative anesthetic considerations during the COVID-19 surge

Material	Environmental	Personnel
Personal protective equipment: consolidated to a single station under direct supervision 24/7 to minimize theft	COVID-19 designated OR	Most anesthesia personnel deployed in ICUs and airway teams
Reuse of N95 masks until soiled or damaged	Preoperative and postoperative units combined	
HMEF used on all cases regardless of COVID-19 status		
Supply carts removed from OR and covered with plastic drape		
All anticipated medications kept in the room and discarded between cases (including emergency medications)		

inspiratory and the expiratory limbs. However, the manufacturer could not guarantee efficacy in preventing viral contamination of the anesthesia machine at the time of the COVID-19 surge at NYP. Another potential point of contamination was the end-tidal CO_2 side-stream modules, which sample gas at the circuit's Y-piece. Similarly, the manufacturers of our machines (GE, Drager) were unable to guarantee prevention of viral contamination. Consequently, we used heat moisture exchangers with integrated filters (HMEF) connected to the endotracheal tube (ETT) on every patient during the initial phases of the COVID-19 surge (**Fig. 1**). This barrier increased airway resistance and added dead space (more relevant for ICU patients; additional discussion later in the ORICU section). By May, manufacturers confirmed through independent testing that the $Etco_2$ module filters prevented SARS-CoV-2 transmission, and the HMEF was moved to the expiratory limb. Months later, King Systems confirmed the efficacy of their built-in filters, and currently, we do not use additional viral filters on our anesthesia circuits.

Aerosol-generating procedures were considered high risk for transmission of SARS-CoV-2, including intubation and extubation, which are common procedures for patients undergoing anesthesia (particularly in emergency surgery). Our intubation strategy is discussed in greater detail later in the airway section. Our extubation strategy included extubating over a face-tent connected to suction or using a Plexiglas box (see Airway section); although far from precise, it was thought that this low-risk additional step was worth attempting to reduce airborne spread of the virus.

Airway Management

At NYP-Columbia, the Department of Anesthesiology staffs an airway team that responds to all emergency intubations and cardiac arrests outside of the emergency room and ICUs, as well as difficult airways anywhere throughout the hospital. This team comprises 1 attending anesthesiologist and 2 resident physicians. Our major adaptations are summarized in **Tables 2** and **3**, with further discussion in the later paragraphs.

Before the COVID-19 surge in NYC, the number of airway activations varied from day to day, but typically remained in the single digits over a 24-hour period. At the

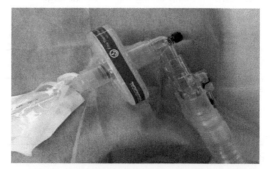

Fig. 1. HMEF use on anesthesia machines. Initially it was unclear if the filters on the CO_2 sampling line and inspiratory/expiratory limbs of the circuits would protect the machine from SARS-CoV-2 contamination. The use of HMEF with confirmed filtration of viral particles at the level of the ETT-circuit connection prevented contamination and is shown here. As manufacturers completed their individual testing, the protocol changed, as the HMEF was moved first to the expiratory limb and then removed entirely (when the CO_2 sampling filter and then circuit filters were confirmed to prevent contamination).

Table 2
Airway and cardiac arrest team considerations during the COVID-19 surge

Material	Environmental	Personnel
PPE backpack (containing contact/droplet/isolation PPE for 2 anesthesia providers)	"Procedure rooms": negative pressure rooms dedicated to intubation	Specific COVID-19 intubation protocol
Portable video laryngoscopes		Creation of a second airway response team to meet volume demands
Aerosol boxes, ultimately not used frequently		Cardiac arrest simulations with medicine, nursing, and respiratory therapy
		Donning and doffing education videos and simulations
		Limiting personnel in room
		PPE observer role created for cardiac arrest

height of the surge, 30 intubations per day were carried out by the Department of Anesthesiology. This increased volume required the creation of a second airway team, the "nonemergency intubation" team. Unlike the traditional airway team, which is activated to a location via pager and overhead announcement, this team was contacted in the same manner as a consult service and was used for patients who needed intubation but were deemed stable enough to wait for at least an hour (for example, a patient who was fatiguing from increased work of breathing but was not imminently desaturating). Close communication and coordination between the 2 airway teams allowed us to triage the urgency of intubations to ensure optimal patient care.

We adjusted our approach to intubation in several ways to minimize the risk of transmission to HCWs. Because the highest risk of aerosol generation was thought to be the actual intubation procedure, NYP-Columbia initially established multiple negative pressure rooms that were dedicated as "procedure rooms." When medically possible, patients who were not already in a negative-pressure room would be moved into these rooms for intubation and subsequently transferred to an ICU once they were intubated and on a closed circuit with a transport ventilator. We further minimized risk by only sending the smallest number of staff in the room during the procedure itself: after all the appropriate equipment was set up, only 2 or 3 HCWs were in the room for induction, intubation, and connection to the ventilator. Backup staff members donned PPE and were available immediately outside the door for additional support in the setting of difficult intubation or hemodynamic instability. We also aimed to minimize time from induction to intubation in order to reduce HCW exposure: our department's policy was that the most experienced clinician on the team would be first to perform laryngoscopy (typically this meant the attending physician). To minimize aerosol generation associated with mask ventilation, rapid sequence intubation was the default approach. We performed video laryngoscopy by default, with the rationale that video laryngoscopy increased the physical distance from the patient's oropharynx. The portability and ease of sanitation of handheld devices over video laryngoscopes with a separate screen proved advantageous as well. Once the ETT was placed, the HMEF was connected and the ETT cuff was inflated before any ventilation to

Table 3
Novel intensive care unit considerations

Material	Environmental	Personnel
Personal protective equipment: consolidated to a single station under direct supervision 24/7 to minimize theft	ICU workspace: computers, pharmacy-dispensing stations, code carts, airway equipment, standard ICU supplies in carts/shelving units, communication boards, central monitoring, point-of-care blood analysis system, personal protective equipment	Tiered staffing model
Ventilators: anesthesia machines used due to shortage, with occasional limitations requiring backup ICU ventilators available	Patient rooms: HEPA-negative air machines, vital signs monitors, ventilators, data jacks, power outlets, gas supply (O_2 and room air), and a large volume of IV pumps, storage, and equipment shelving units	Significant investment in education: direct teaching, in-servicing, layers of supervision (both MD and RN), daily briefings, infographics, protocols
Drug shortages	Line-of-sight limited in novel spaces; requiring additional precautions for audio and visual alarms/assessments	Identification of areas of staffing shortage and creation of separate teams to address these limitations in patient care (eg, anesthesia helping fill traditional respiratory therapy roles)
	Pharmacy supply chain	Protocolization of care in general, with close ICU provider oversight for specialized management

rapidly establish a closed circuit to minimize viral contamination. When feasible, ventilation was immediately established by directly connecting to the ventilator to minimize the number of circuit disconnects.

We designed a system of PPE backpacks that the anesthesia clinicians would take to airway emergencies and cardiac arrests (**Fig. 2**). The PPE backpacks contained N95 masks, surgical masks, eye protection, fluid-proof isolation gowns (in contrast to the standard gowns used at NYP for contact isolation, which is only fluid resistant), extralong gloves in various sizes to ensure full coverage at the forearms, bouffant caps (not routinely stocked in isolation carts pre–COVID-19), and extra video laryngoscope blade covers. The backpacks were plastic rather than fabric to facilitate cleaning. These backpacks were sanitized and restocked in between uses and stored in a locked room only accessible to department personnel.

We used plastic aerosol boxes with similar design as reported in the literature.[3] These transparent boxes offered another layer between the patient and HCW to contain droplets and possibly aerosols. We trialed this equipment first in our simulation center and then for direct patient care. In anecdotal experience, use of the aerosol boxes appeared to increase intubation time and hypoxemic events; thus, we

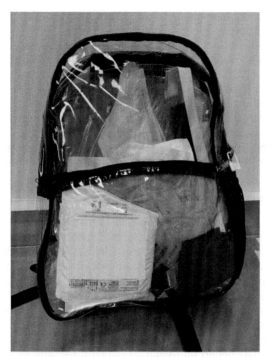

Fig. 2. PPE backpack. Each bag contained HEPA filter, N95 masks (small and regular size), face shields, video laryngoscope blade covers, isolation gowns (waterproof), sterile gown, bouffant hats, beard cover, sterile gloves, and biohazard bag (for used video laryngoscope).

ultimately thought that the harms outweighed the potential benefits for routine use during intubation. The efficacy of this style of aerosol box in reducing HCW exposure has since been called into question.[4] We continued to use the device for extubation, which is less technically complex and therefore has fewer downsides.

Cardiac arrest management required specific considerations. Prepandemic, cardiac arrest activations at our institution often resulted in more than a dozen HCWs crowding into a patient room, often neglecting isolation precautions. Given the increased concerns for minimizing HCW exposure as well as conserving PPE, we created a new role of "Observer/Relay Provider." This role, typically filled by the charge nurse or patient care director, was primarily dedicated to standing by the door to personally confirm adequate donning and doffing procedures, to limit the number of HCWs to the bare minimum necessary for safe patient care, and to act as the point person for communication/equipment transport in and out of the rooms. After these protocols were formalized, we designed a cardiac arrest simulation and then hosted multidisciplinary sessions to reinforce education with internal medicine, nursing, and rapid response teams. Videos were recorded and distributed for further education.

OBSTETRIC ANESTHESIA

The Obstetric Anesthesiology Division at NYP-Columbia faced a different set of challenges but followed the same general principles of ensuring safe patient care while minimizing HCW exposure to SARS-CoV-2. The patient volume was unchanged because of the nature of the obstetric population. Aerosol generation during intubation/extubation was considered the highest risk; therefore, early neuraxial labor analgesia was strongly encouraged for all parturients. If necessary and unavoidable, general anesthesia and intubation were performed as described above in the airway management section. Even in March when the availability of polymerase chain reaction testing was still limited, the obstetric population was deemed high priority in the NYP system given the high risk for HCW exposure during emergency aerosol-generating procedures. Consequently, preadmission testing was performed on all labor and delivery patients, and this information was invaluable in ensuring proper isolation precautions were maintained. More in-depth discussion about the NYP-Columbia Obstetric Anesthesiology Division's response has been written elsewhere.[5]

OPERATING ROOM INTENSIVE CARE UNIT

At NYP-Columbia, the baseline ICU capacity is 117 beds across 8 discrete units. During the COVID-19 surge, we had a peak of more than 220 ICU patients. To meet the rapidly growing demand for ICU beds and ventilators, we created several novel ICUs over the course of weeks. The Department of Anesthesiology was primarily involved in the conversion of 23 unused ORs into an ORICU. The plan for an ORICU had strategic advantages: ventilators were running low quickly and the anesthesia machines were unused given the lack of elective surgery. In addition, given the anesthesia machines' large size, it seemed logical to convert the relatively large OR rooms into multiple bed ICU rooms.

Planning for ORICU began on March 21, when it became clear that the patient burden would rapidly overwhelm the standard ICU capacity, and within 2 days, the ORICU began accepting its first patients. The original plan was to admit low-acuity intubated patients from traditional ICUs. Specifically, patients requiring renal replacement therapy or experiencing severe hemodynamic instability were thought to be better suited for a traditional ICU. This approach lasted for less than a week before the large volume of ICU admissions required accepting patients to whichever bed was open, regardless of unit. The ORICU was active from March 24 through May 14 and cared for 133 patients in total.

The ORICU comprised 7 pods. A pod was a cluster of 3 or 4 ORs linked to a single sterile core. Most pods could treat 12 patients except for Pod G, which was a single room with a capacity of 6 patients (**Fig. 3**). Each sterile core conceptualized a self-sufficient ICU space with all necessary equipment: computers, pharmacy dispensing stations, code carts, airway equipment, standard ICU supplies in carts/shelving units, communication boards, central monitoring, point-of-care blood analysis system, and PPE. Additional equipment was stored in unused OR stockrooms as well as the PACU. These cores were also the primary points of entry/exit to the ORs to minimize foot traffic; the standard OR doors were only used for patient transport and otherwise kept locked. Although the ORs themselves were meticulously maintained with contact/droplet/airborne precautions, HCWs doffed their isolation gowns and gloves as they exited an OR but maintained droplet/airborne precautions in the core.

Each OR in the ORICU was converted to treat 3 to 4 patients, typically limited by physical space or gas access (**Fig. 4**). The first step in the conversion was the addition of HEPA negative air machines that converted the rooms from positive pressure to negative. After that, structural changes included additional vital signs monitors, ventilators, data jacks, power outlets, gas supply (both O_2 and room air), and a large volume of intravenous (IV) pumps (typically 6 per patient, given the need for prolonged sedation, vasoactive medications, and antibiotics). The layout of each room led to

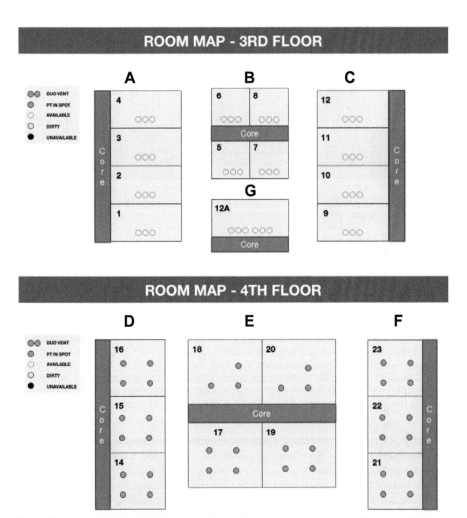

Fig. 3. Floor map of the ORICU. Each of 7 sterile cores was repurposed into an ICU work-space and connected to 3 to 4 ORs, each hosting 3 to 4 ventilated patients.

restricted visibility: unlike a standard ICU, which is designed to maintain line of sight, the ORICU only had 2 small windows into each OR from the sterile cores. Consequently, the rooms had to be arranged so vital signs, ventilators, and patients were facing these windows. Even still, these structural barriers provided a significant challenge as the numbers and alerts were often too small to be readily seen from the core. As an additional challenge, the heavy doors in the OR and the loud fans used for negative pressure made hearing alarms difficult. These visibility and structural issues were partially ameliorated by configuring the ventilator alarms to transmit to the central monitor station and installing cameras (intended for monitoring infants in the home) in the rooms. Despite these modifications, audiovisual problems persisted up until the closing of the ORICU.

At the time of the COVID-19 surge, ventilators were in short supply. Consequently, anesthesia machines (Drager, Datex-Ohmeda, and GE machines are in use at NYP-Columbia) were used as ICU ventilators for most patients in the ORICU. This was

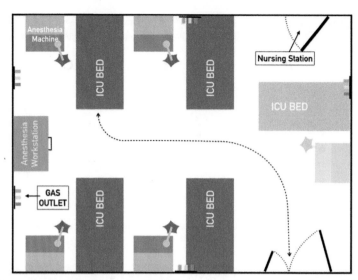

Fig. 4. Representative layout of a single ORICU room. This is one of the larger ORs and was able to hold 4 ventilated ICU patients. We followed 2 guiding principles for the room layout: 1. The beds and anesthesia machines had to be positioned close to a wall or beam-mounted gas outlets and data jacks (one per patient); 2. The patient had to be accessible from both sides of the bed; 3. The arrangement had to allow for each patient to be moved out of the room without other beds or equipment needing rearrangement, as most patients were severely ill. Each room had 1 anesthesia workstation containing emergency equipment and medicines for resuscitation. The light-colored bed and anesthesia machine on the right represent the possibility to extend capacity to 5 beds in case of increasing demand.

associated with several problems. First, the anesthesia machine maximum alarm volume was quieter than a standard ICU ventilator, as alluded to above. Second, the different handling and interface made the management more challenging; nursing and respiratory therapy were not familiar with the machines, requiring more direct anesthesia provider supervision during routine care (eg, increasing Fio_2 before turning a patient). Third, the anesthesia machines do not have built-in inspiratory and expiratory hold maneuvers to easily assess plateau pressures and intrinsic PEEP. Fourth, CO_2 absorbers were quickly saturated and needed frequent exchange. High gas flow rates were used (>15 L per minute) to minimize absorbent consumption as well as reduce moisture buildup in the HMEF, which increased resistance when fully saturated; this created the additional concern that we would exceed the hospital's central oxygen supply, which was addressed with biomedical and facilities departments. Finally, the anesthesia machines were unable to maintain adequate ventilation at the extremes of care: for the sickest patients with the worst compliance and highest respiratory rate, often the anesthesia machine would fail to deliver set volumes and the patient would need to be switched to an ICU ventilator (Puritan Bennett 840, LTV-1200, or Maquet Servo-U are all in use at NYP-Columbia). Consequently, 2 ICU ventilators were kept on standby in the event of inadequate ventilation, although the anesthesia machines were adequate for most patients.

The pharmacy division faced many challenges as well. From a logistical standpoint, doubling the ICU capacity meant supply chain issues, as these new ICUs all had to be restocked aggressively; this was especially true in late March and early April, when the vast majority of patients were deeply sedated for ventilation purposes. Furthermore, this high demand led to medication shortages. These shortages were addressed by our pharmacy team through twice-daily communications with ORICU leadership. For example, midazolam was briefly on shortage, so patients were switched to lorazepam, diazepam, or even chlordiazepoxide until the division could replenish their supply. Similar rotations occurred with fentanyl and hydromorphone. Overall, close communication allowed for adjustment of sedation agents with enough advance notice to educate clinicians on how to use less familiar medications, ensuring safe patient care in the face of significant resource limitation.

The staffing model required continuous iterative evaluation. Our model was based on the SCCM tiered staffing strategy[6] (https://www.sccm.org/Blog/March-2020/United-States-Resource-Availability-for-COVID-19), but needed adjustment for the staffing limitations experienced at NYP-Columbia (**Fig. 5**). First, there was a significant shortage of critical care nurses (CCRNs) and respiratory therapists (RTs). Many tasks were explicitly shared between nurses and medical clinicians, such as administering medications to help assist the non–ICU-trained nurses as they were thrust into an ICU nursing role. The available CCRNs were further prioritized for a "resource" role, which was more supervisory and focused on providing nursing assistance where needed. This model of shared responsibilities and increased supervision allowed for the flexibility needed to fill gaps experience and coverage. The Medical ICU nursing team established a portable prone team that could prone patients in any ICU (before the pandemic, prone positioning for ARDS could only be used in the Medical ICU). Formal nursing education efforts also occurred throughout the duration of the surge

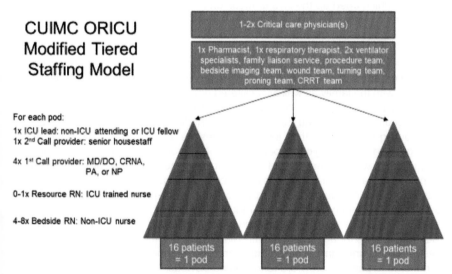

CUIMC ORICU Modified Tiered Staffing Model

1-2x Critical care physician(s)

1x Pharmacist, 1x respiratory therapist, 2x ventilator specialists, family liaison service, procedure team, bedside imaging team, wound team, turning team, proning team, CRRT team

For each pod:

1x ICU lead: non-ICU attending or ICU fellow
1x 2nd Call provider: senior housestaff

4x 1st Call provider: MD/DO, CRNA, PA, or NP

0-1x Resource RN: ICU trained nurse

4-8x Bedside RN: Non-ICU nurse

16 patients = 1 pod   16 patients = 1 pod   16 patients = 1 pod

Fig. 5. CUIMC ORICU modified tiered staffing model. Based on the SCCM tiered staffing mode, adapted to meet our specific staffing needs. One to 2 critical care physicians provided oversight to 3 pods. Each pod of 16 patients was staffed by 1 "ICU lead" filling the traditional ICU attending role, 1 "second call provider" filling the senior resident/fellow role, 4 "first call providers" filling the APP/resident role, and a variable number of nurses depending on staffing availability. The largest modification to the SCCM model is seen in the large gray box in the middle: the many limitations (resource, skill, time, or knowledge) experienced during the COVID-19 surge necessitated the creation of many specialized ancillary teams to fill particularly challenging aspects of ICU care. CRNA, certified registered nurse anesthetist; NP, nurse practitioner; PA, physician assistant.

with dramatic effects. For example, dedicated wound care and turn teams focused primarily on teaching the non–ICU-trained nurses in addition to direct patient care, which ultimately had the effect of rapidly increasing competence of the ORICU nursing team.

Similarly, NYP-Columbia experienced a shortage of RTs during the surge. This, coupled with unfamiliarity with the anesthesia machines, necessitated the creation of the "anesthesia ventilator specialist" role. This role was filled by residents and attendings. The ventilator specialist team rounded on all ORICU patients at least twice a day and responded to any ventilator issues throughout the shift. Responsibilities included maintenance of the anesthesia machine (including assessing the need to exchange HMEFs and CO_2 absorbers), adjusting ventilator settings following the ARDSnet protocol, checking plateau and intrinsic PEEP, documentation, and performing typical respiratory interventions, such as delivering nebulized medications and performing endotracheal suctioning/lavage. Although a necessary step in minimizing contamination, the use of HMEF on all patients in the ORICU was particularly challenging for this team. When dry, the HMEF added minimally to airway resistance. However, when they became fully saturated, peak airway pressures were significantly increased by as much as 10 to 15 cm H_2O, often resulting in ventilation failure. Exchanging HMEFs became one of the first steps in troubleshooting high airway pressure alarms. Checking plateau pressures and intrinsic PEEP required specific education and protocolization because our anesthesia machines lack inspiratory and expiratory hold maneuvers. By investing effort into devising education and protocols with RT input, our anesthesia team quickly became facile with routine respiratory therapy tasks, which freed up the RTs to focus on more acute or complex management.

Because NYP-Columbia has a large roster of physicians and because elective procedures and outpatient clinics were on hold, the ORICU had access to many skilled clinicians. Most of the anesthesia and surgical residents worked as first- and second-call providers. Anesthesiologists in our department who were immunocompromised or elderly formed a Family Liaison Service that served as the primary point of contact with the family as well as facilitated goals of care conversations, freeing up the primary ICU clinicians to focus on clinical care. The Family Liaison Service was able to secure iPads through donations and scheduled video calls with patient families, allowing them to see their loved ones despite the limited visitation throughout the surge. The psychological impact of complete isolation of the patients from any family member was unprecedented and substantial; therefore, the Family Liaison Service proved to be essential in limiting the emotional stress and despair. Dermatologists joined the wound care team. Radiologists formed a point-of-care ultrasound team that was invaluable as echocardiology and radiology technicians were also understaffed to meet the surge in demand. Surgeons and interventional radiologists formed a bedside procedure service for arterial line, central line, and chest tube placement.[7] These services required significant communication and troubleshooting but paid off quickly, as the benefits to patient care were tangible and obvious.

The educational aspect was particularly important with the pandemic staffing model, where ICU attending physicians provided oversight to several non-ICU attending physicians and therefore could not round on every patient. This process was made easier by the relatively homogenous patient population, that is, everyone had the same primary disease process, which allowed us to protocolize key aspects of our management, particularly regarding sedation and ventilator support. Once these protocols were established, we adopted a multimedia approach to disseminating this information. Brief teaching sessions were held before rounds daily; infographics with key take-home points were hung in the cores, and printouts, such as rounding templates and protocols, were distributed to the staff (**Fig. 6**). Throughout the course of the ORICU, more than 100 guidelines, protocols, and infographics were generated. Through continued emphasis on education and quality improvement, the anesthesia department was able to ensure a high standard of care was delivered despite considerable variability in provider ICU experience.

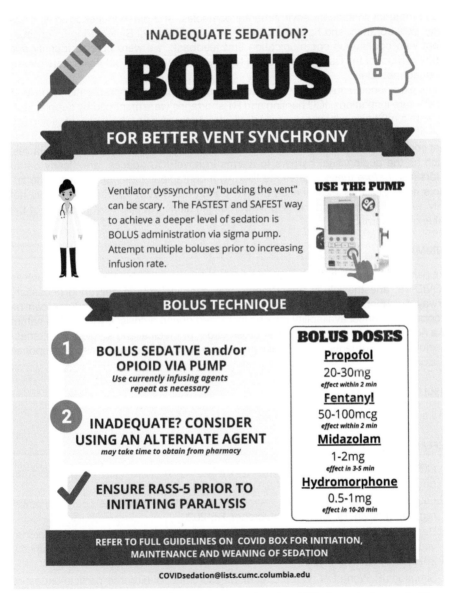

Fig. 6. Example infographic used for patient care education. With the redeployment of hundreds of non-ICU and nonanesthesia providers into ICU roles, rapid education was a priority. Sedation was particularly challenging in the ORICU patients given the additional physical barriers to both detecting and treating inadequate sedation.

DISCUSSION

The anesthesiologists at NYP played a key role during the COVID-19 pandemic, as the disease spread like wildfire throughout NYC during March 2020, quickly overwhelming health care systems. Throughout this, perioperative services were maintained and adapted to a novel disease with limited testing and unknown management; the airway and cardiac arrest teams were stretched beyond their usual capacity, and novel ICU spaces were rapidly established to accommodate the influx of critically ill patients. We faced material limitations, environmental obstacles, and personnel shortages; creativity, collaboration, and hard work were the only constants. By fostering an environment with continuous communication and feedback, we were able to identify and address most of the issues that arose. However, many of these solutions were merely stopgap measures.

Our experience highlights the need for a thoughtful pandemic preparation plan at all health care institutions. ICU nursing and RT shortages were managed by supplementing with a multidisciplinary team fully dedicated to the mission; however, "training up" non-ICU providers as well as recruiting experienced personnel is a lengthy process that could have started months earlier. Similarly, many of the environmental obstacles, such as the audio/visual barriers to alarms in novel ICU spaces, are clearly better addressed *before* these spaces are filled with contagious patients. As such, the authors hope that their experiences at NYP during the COVID-19 pandemic serve not only as a reference for addressing resource limitations but also as a reminder of the value of preparation.

SUMMARY

In a pandemic, particularly one with predominant respiratory disease patterns, such as COVID-19, anesthesiology departments play a critical role in delivering necessary airway management and ventilation support. Because elective procedures can be stopped, personnel availability may be increased during a crisis. Owing to the nature of a hospital-based specialty at the "crossroads" of medical and surgical care, anesthesiology departments are well positioned to be central players in a hospital response to a crisis.

DISCLOSURE

The authors have nothing to disclose.

REFERENCES

1. COVID-19: Data. Available at: https://www1.nyc.gov/site/doh/covid/covid-19-data.page. Accessed October 28, 2020.
2. Latest News on COVID-19. Available at: https://columbiasurgery.org/news/regarding-covid-19. Accessed October 28, 2020.
3. Begley JL, Lavery KE, Nickson CP, et al. The aerosol box for intubation in coronavirus disease 2019 patients: an in-situ simulation crossover study. Anaesthesia 2020;75(8):1014–21.
4. Simpson JP, Wong DN, Verco L, et al. Measurement of airborne particle exposure during simulated tracheal intubation using various proposed aerosol containment devices during the COVID-19 pandemic. Anaesthesia 2020;75(12):1587–95.
5. Bauer ME, Bernstein K, Dinges E, et al. Obstetric anesthesia during the COVID-19 pandemic. Anesth Analgesia 2020;131(1):7–15.

6. United States resource availability for COVID-19. Available at: https://www.sccm. org/Blog/March-2020/United-States-Resource-Availability-for-COVID-19. Accessed October 28, 2020.
7. Coons BE, Tam SF, Okochi S. Rapid development of resident-led procedural response teams to support patient care during the coronavirus disease 2019 epidemic: a surgical workforce activation team. JAMA Surg 2020;155(8):683–4.

Clinical Research Redirection and Optimization During a Pandemic

Ludmilla Candido Santos, MD[a], Ying Hui Low, MD[b],
Konstantin Inozemtsev, MD[c], Alexander Nagrebetsky, MD, MSc[b],*

KEYWORDS

- Pandemic • COVID-19 • Research limitations • Optimization • Publication surge

KEY POINTS

- Pandemics create acute strains on research resources.
- Research challenges presented by past/current pandemics are similar in nature.
- High demand for information in the setting of a pandemic may decrease the average quality of scientific publications.
- We discuss recommendations for future research, during this public health crisis and others.

INTRODUCTION AND HISTORY

The first diagnosis in the United States of severe acute respiratory syndrome coronavirus 2 (SARS-CoV-2), also known as coronavirus disease (COVID-19) (which is how this virus is referred to henceforth), was received on January 20, 2020.[1,2] On March 18, 2020, the United States Food and Drug Administration (FDA) issued an updated guideline for the conduct of clinical trials, which highlighted the need to adhere to social distancing and quarantine guidelines.[3] Most research activities in major institutions were suspended soon after that, despite the need for scientific research to address the pandemic.

Past pandemics, such as the severe acute respiratory syndrome coronavirus (SARs-CoV-1) in 2002; H1N1 influenza in 2009; Middle East respiratory syndrome, which started in 2012 and is still lingering; and Ebola virus in 2019, have seen a deficient response in clinical research.[4] Inadequate research collaboration and funding,

L.C. Santos and Y.H. Low contributed equally to the work.
[a] Emergency Medicine Network, Massachusetts General Hospital, Harvard Medical School, 55 Fruit Street, Boston, MA 02114, USA; [b] Department of Anesthesia, Critical Care and Pain Medicine, Massachusetts General Hospital, Harvard Medical School, 55 Fruit Street, Boston, MA 02114, USA; [c] Department of Anesthesiology, Dartmouth-Hitchcock Medical Center, One Medical Center Drive, Lebanon, NH 03756, USA
* Corresponding author.
E-mail address: anagrebetsky@mgh.harvard.edu

Anesthesiology Clin 39 (2021) 379–388
https://doi.org/10.1016/j.anclin.2021.03.004
1932-2275/21/© 2021 Elsevier Inc. All rights reserved.

anesthesiology.theclinics.com

particularly in vulnerable regions, have been identified in a previous review.[5] In its contemplation of lessons learned from the historical inquiry of pandemic mitigation strategies, the Institute of Medicine[6] observes that progress in clinical research, particularly with surveillance, rapid communications, modern computing, and epidemic modeling, has the potential to not only mitigate but prevent future pandemics.

The goal of this article is to explore and summarize the effects of pandemics on clinical research and to explore approaches to effectively redirect and optimize clinical research in future pandemics. The discussion is limited to observational and interventional studies in clinical research; basic science research is beyond the scope of this article.

DISCUSSION
Effects of Pandemics on Components of Clinical Research

The components of any modern research framework are familiar to all scientists and can be classified broadly into the following steps: (1) generating a research hypothesis and developing a study protocol; (2) obtaining regulatory approval; (3) studying implementation, including securing adequate funding for completion of all study processes, such as interventions and data collection; and (4) analysis and publication of data in the form of a article.[7,8] Public health emergencies of a new pandemic create acute strains in resources that often affect critical elements of executing a research protocol. These are discussed and summarized in **Table 1**.

Study design
Leading up to the appearance of COVID-19, other infectious disease pandemics and large-scale public health emergencies have been cited as events that highlight the need for a coordinated research response.[9] For instance, the 2009 H1N1 pandemic, 2010 Haiti earthquake, Deepwater Horizon oil spill, and 2011 Fukushima Daiichi nuclear disaster were highlighted as recent events where the acute strains placed on government agencies, including health care and scientific organizations, limited the ability to address key components of research.[9] The authors recommend the assembly of a ready team of experts who can generate relevant research questions and prioritize and monitor research needs.[9] This forms the first step of ensuring conditions for rapid data collection and appropriate human subjects review, mechanisms for rapid funding, and exposure monitoring.[9]

It also is paramount to ensure that research planning is carried out in an ethical manner despite the emerging disaster, by engaging both public and scientific experts to address specific needs of the different communities involved in research. These discussions should address ethical questions that arise during public health emergencies and the risk that research might be perceived as an exploitation of vulnerable people or communities in a state of disaster.[9] Investigators also have underscored the importance of abiding by systematic risk and ethical evaluations when assessing the ethics of pandemic-related research, particularly in high-risk clinical trials, such as early-phase trials of potential vaccines for COVID-19.[10] Such safety considerations has to be balanced deftly with the need for quicker regulatory approval.

Regulatory approval
Even before the current pandemic, investigators have called for the development of more precise consensus guidelines addressing the waiver of informed consent in emergency research.[11] In 2020, the challenges of carrying out emergency research with exceptions for informed consent were highlighted, with some investigators calling

Table 1
Effects of a pandemic on clinical research

Steps in the Research Process	Effects in the Setting of a Pandemic
Study design	
Generating a hypothesis	Lack of expertise in emerging disease Limited expert availability with clinician-scientists responding to high demand in clinical care
Study protocol design	Prioritization of studies that yield quick results rather than long-term outcomes Delays in gathering preliminary data that may help inform main study design (eg, for a power analysis) Difficulty ensuring proper risk and ethics analysis and that research planning is ethical and not seen as an exploitation of vulnerable communities
Regulatory approval	
Institutional board review	Potential for delay with institutional board review and approval
FDA approval	Potential fast-tracking for COVID-19 studies Potential delay for non–COVID-19 studies
Study implementation	
Funding	Allocation of funding toward more immediate health care needs
Intervention delivery and data collection	Site closures Travel limitations Interruptions to supply chain Limited access to research facilities and equipment due to official stay-at-home orders Limited access to the delivery of interventions Disrupted patient screening and recruitment Limited in-person baseline and follow-up data collection
Data review and publication	
Data analysis	Redirection of resources to pandemic-related projects Disrupted work environment and team dynamics due to remote work settings
Article writing and review	Perceived pressure to produce results Decreased peer review standards due to high demand for information Potential impact on quality of publications

for the need to offer appropriate means for rapid consultation to support such exceptions.[12]

In addition, investigators observed the need for greater regulatory flexibility during pandemics to manage both the goals of protecting participants and promoting the development of high-quality evidence that informs patient care during the pandemic.[12] Although many institutional review boards (IRBs) also took steps to speed the review of COVID-19 protocols, this led to a challenge of heightened workload and personal responsibilities for IRB members, particularly at academic institutions, and may not be sustainable.[12]

Furthermore, the traditional safeguards for research that involves incarcerated persons, which was a population of patients heavily impacted by COVID-19, possibly may be to their detriment, and investigators have suggested the need to allow such research when there is the prospect of direct benefit to these individuals in custody.[12]

During COVID-19, the FDA also helped conduct ultrarapid protocol reviews for research subject to investigational new drug and investigational device exemption requirements, as part of the Coronavirus Treatment Acceleration Program.[13]

Study implementation

The inaccessibility of trial participants and research personnel due to social distancing rules during COVID-19 led to delays in patient enrollment, and operational gaps in clinical trials may have a negative impact on data integrity.[14]

Patient screening and recruitment. The success and generalizability of clinical trials depend considerably on extensive participant enrollment.[15] During COVID-19, patient recruitment and ease of conducting in-person visits were significantly affected, not only by official policy limiting nonessential movement but also by fears of a poorly characterized disease among participants and caregivers.[15,16]

Consent process. With isolation or physical distancing requirements, the FDA recommended the use of electronic consent via the COVID MyStudies mobile device application or the use of phone or videoconferencing. A comprehensive discussion with a potential study participant, however, is time consuming—for instance, the discussion of every possible alternative to enrollment in a given COVID-19 protocol, particularly in the early phases of a pandemic, when available alternatives were rapidly changing. It has been suggested that regulations be revised to allow more flexibility for only context-appropriate disclosures to patients.[12]

Intervention delivery and data collection. COVID-19 resulted in extensive travel restrictions and site closures, in addition to the diversion of nonessential hospital space, including research areas, to enhance patient isolation.[17] Investigators also have to consider the relative risks and benefits of conducting research activities and provide a safe environment and, where appropriate, reassurance to participants.[16] In addition, disruption of supply chains for investigational drugs further jeopardized delivery of study interventions.[17] Protocols often required modification to ensure adherence to intervention and measurement of outcomes, including remote data collection by telephone, video or telehealth platforms, and carrying out follow-up testing at home where possible.[18,19] Other than transitioning to remote operations, where possible, the pandemic experience also has highlighted the value of research networks—established pathways for sharing information between sites can help speed up the process of gathering valuable data and may overcome obstacles, such as those encountered during the current pandemic.[19]

Data review and publication

A step in the research process that may seem unhindered by the COVID-19 pandemic is the publication of articles, although it remains debatable whether this is a marker of research success. It may be contended that even prior to the pandemic, publication was a process carried out entirely remotely, so it was least affected by the new pandemic rules.

This apparent success in COVID-19 research, however, is marred by the following criticisms. First, the number of publications also appears to be heavily inflated by non–peer-reviewed or nonoriginal research, such as editorials and opinion articles, many of which are cited later. Second, the publication and visibility of potentially impactful non—COVID-19 articles may be affected by the overwhelming demand for COVID-19 research.

Publication Surge

As illustrated in **Fig. 1**, the number of publications on COVID-19 was unparalleled. For comparison, after 6 months of the report of the first case of SARS-CoV-1 in February 2003,[20] 929 articles had been published as situation unfolded; and by the sixth month after the 2009 pandemic of H1N1 Influenza started, 1245 articles about the virus were available on PubMed-indexed journals. By contrast, in June 2020, the number of articles published on COVID-19 was approximately 30-times higher (35,891) than in the previous pandemics.[21–23]

The average quality of early COVID-19 publications, however, was met with harsh critique among the both scientific and journalism communities, for the peer review step frequently was skipped in a fast-tracking publication process.[21–23] This pandemic also saw many investigators using preprint servers to disseminate their work.[24] These servers, such as medRxiv, sponsored by Yale University, have become popular sources of information among journalists. Some journals, as *The Lancet*, also make preprints available to the public, and, despite containing a disclaimer that these are articles that have not completed the peer review process or been accepted,[25] they have been used as references by journalists who are looking for the latest updates on COVID-19.[26,27] Multiple preprints on COVID-19 that have been covered by popular media on COVID-19 have been written and retracted within the same year.[28]

Although preprints and articles on preliminary results are much criticized, there are arguments in favor of their utility. Early publication of research methodology and findings allows for earlier detection of methodological issues by the readers. Publication of preliminary results may allow younger, less established researchers to disseminate their ideas and data without having to subject themselves to prohibitive criticism from reviewers of well-known journals, while still receiving credits for their efforts.

These potential benefits, however, must be weighed against the risk of low-quality, non–peer-reviewed research fueling media-driven panic or resulting in inappropriate clinical and policy decisions based on erroneous data, which both could cause harm to individuals and compromise scientific integrity.[29–32]

Even articles published in reputable journals have been retracted, including from *Annals of Internal Medicine*,[33] *The Lancet*,[34,35] and *The New England Journal of Medicine*.[36] A recent review reports that, despite the large number of publications, only a fraction of the published studies fulfilled the principles of evidence-based practice.[37]

The publication onslaught also may reflect a prioritization of studies that yield quick results rather than long-term outcomes. Other investigators also have called for

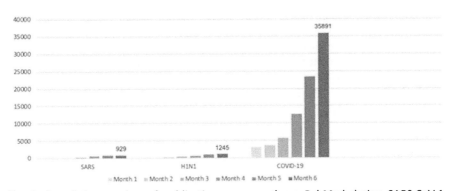

Fig. 1. Cumulative number of publications per month on PubMed during SARS-CoV-1, H1N1, and COVID-19 outbreaks as of August 28, 2020.

researchers to collaborate in larger high-quality investigations, rather than duplicate research in multiple small trials with analogous hypotheses, which may be easier to carry out but less likely to yield precise results.[32]

Concurrent Non–COVID-19 Research

As discussed previously, a veritable explosion of COVID-19 related trials, now numbering in the thousands, represents a significant shift in scientific effort and energy expenditure.[38] Other key basic and clinical research endeavors have been stymied or halted by mandatory facility shutdowns, staff quarantine and distancing measures, suspension of animal and human clinical trials, and loss or reallocation of funding.[39]

In addition to serving as a significant setback for scientific innovation itself, this has had a negative impact on several patients without COVID-19, including many in vulnerable populations, such as those receiving cancer care and immunosuppressive therapy.[40] Many were participating or expecting enrollment in clinical trials, a significant proportion of which was suspended or halted altogether[41] or had recruitment drop precipitously.[42]

Withdrawal of funding from critical research should be avoided or limited whenever possible due to its long-term ramifications for both affected patients, and the scientific community at large. Importantly, ongoing work in related fields may elucidate underlying mechanisms of pathogenesis and treatment of COVID-19 itself, and vice versa.[43]

Research Redirection and Collaboration

With a bevy of researchers addressing the topic from multiple angles, there also has been a growing concern over studies being inadequately powered and suffering from redundancy and heterogeneity in methodology and outcome measurement. As such, there is a need for coordination and establishment of clear guidelines for research and reporting.[44]

Several international consortia, including diverse specialty groups[45] and global health organizations,[46] have offered core outcome sets for trials pertinent to COVID-19. At minimum, these core outcomes should be addressed to maximize data utility and facilitate international collaboration and data pooling efforts.

To encourage international collaboration further, a group of National Science and Technology Advisors spanning numerous countries issued a call to publishers to make COVID-19 publications and associated data freely available in the public domain,[47] highlighting the importance of information and data sharing as means of increasing scientific yield and building more robust data sets for current and future clinical trials.[48]

Furthermore, as research efforts begin bearing fruit, several important differences in symptomatology, complications, and burden of disease within and between populations have emerged. Following the initial paucity of information, geographic, genetic, gender-based, racial, cultural, and socioeconomic variations, among others, have demonstrated important and sometimes drastic differences with significant implications for both treatment and preventative measures.[49]

Research Optimization

As more data emerge, attention must shift from simply examining comparative epidemiology to utilizing it to guide further research needs, address contributing inequities, and help protect those groups and populations that emerge as most vulnerable.[50] At the same time, carefully controlling for a maximal number of such variables during subgroup analysis serves to eliminate spurious correlations and maximize generalizability, crucial to both informed clinical decisions and policy making.[51]

Some of the obstacles posed by the pandemic also can be overcome by enhancing collaborative efforts between researchers, for instance, in the form of data registries. National societies frequently have the capacity to facilitate and coordinate research efforts. For example, the American Society of Anesthesiologists Committee on Critical Care Medicine has served as a platform for networking and site recruitment for the COVID-19 ICU Registry. The COVID-19 ICU Registry[52] is a multi-institutional and international collaboration to collect critical care and respiratory data about patients with COVID-19, with the goals of being able to identify key risk factors for severe illness and disease patterns and potentially to assess treatment efficacy. The CORAL series of studies[53] is another example of a multicenter effort to collect and share data between tens of institutions nationwide.

Health care workers themselves appear to be at elevated risk for contracting the disease, and the intubateCOVID registry, which was designed to track various aspects and outcomes of airway management of infected patients, demonstrated a notable incidence of COVID-19 symptoms, confirmed infection, and sequelae affecting approximately 10% of intubating staff.[54] This, compounded with health care workers' increased risk of being asymptomatic or presymptomatic carriers[55] capable of transmitting the disease to their families and others,[56] can significantly affect both productivity and attitudes toward remaining clinically and academically active.

SUMMARY

The COVID-19 pandemic has seen many hurdles to crucial research processes, in particular those that depend on personnel interactions, in providing safeguards against the incipient infectious disease. At the same time, there was a rapid redirection of research, driven by popular and social media and demand for pandemic-related content, to the detriment of non–COVID-19 research and perhaps to COVID-19 research itself.

This pandemic has provided critical lessons to the authors, who believe the following will be essential for future research success: (1) regional, national, and global scientific societies need to rapidly identify strategic high-yield areas for research based on preliminary data and coordinate efforts at acquiring reliable quality data from multiple sources for collaborative data analysis, including in the form of data registries; (2) prompt recognition by regulatory authorities of areas of flexibility that are relevant to the new crisis; and (3) publishers should lay out guidelines for what constitutes a significant investigation and help provide a constant source of quality control for the research enthusiasm that comes with a novel research question.

Although there is little motivation to create and update contingency strategies for research coalitions, regulation, and publishing during periods of nonemergency, these efforts are likely to be most successful when preplanned and pretested at a time of relative abundance of resources. It would be prudent for the scientific community to maintain processes learned during COVID-19 so that these lessons do not need to be relearned during the next public health crisis.

ACKNOWLEDGMENTS (FUNDING INFORMATION)

This study is funded by T32 NIH grant: 2T32GM007592-41.

DISCLOSURE

The authors have no conflicts of interest to disclose.

REFERENCES

1. Holshue ML, DeBolt C, Lindquist S, et al. First Case of 2019 Novel Coronavirus in the United States. N Engl J Med 2020;382(10):929–36.
2. Harcourt J, Tamin A, Lu Xea. Severe acute respiratory syndrome coronavirus 2 from patient with coronavirus disease, United States. 2020. Available at: https://wwwnc.cdc.gov/eid/article/26/6/20-0516_article. Accessed October 27, 2020.
3. U.S. Food and Drug Administration. Clinical Trial Conduct During the COVID-19 Pandemic. 2020. Available at: https://www.fda.gov/drugs/coronavirus-covid-19-drugs/clinical-trial-conduct-during-covid-19-pandemic. Accessed October 27, 2020.
4. Rojek AM, Horby PW. Modernising epidemic science: enabling patient-centred research during epidemics. BMC Med 2016;14(1):212.
5. Sigfrid L, Maskell K, Bannister PG, et al. Addressing challenges for clinical research responses to emerging epidemics and pandemics: a scoping review. BMC Med 2020;18(1):190.
6. Institute of Medicine (US). Ethical and Legal Considerations in mitigating pandemic disease: Workshop summary. Washington, DC: The National Academies Press; 2007.
7. Thiese MS. Observational and interventional study design types; an overview. Biochem Med (Zagreb) 2014;24(2):199–210.
8. Eriksen MB, Frandsen TF. The impact of patient, intervention, comparison, outcome (PICO) as a search strategy tool on literature search quality: a systematic review. J Med Libr Assoc 2018;106(4):420–31.
9. Lurie N, Manolio T, Patterson AP, et al. Research as a part of public health emergency response. N Engl J Med 2013;368(13):1251–5.
10. Bull S, Jamrozik E, Binik A, et al. SARS-CoV-2 challenge studies: ethics and risk minimisation [published online ahead of print, 2020 Sep 25]. J Med Ethics 2020. https://doi.org/10.1136/medethics-2020-106504. medethics-2020-106504.
11. Vaslef SN, Cairns CB, Falletta JM. Ethical and regulatory challenges associated with the exception from informed consent requirements for emergency research: from experimental design to institutional review board approval. Arch Surg 2006; 141(10):1019–23 [discussion: 1024].
12. Fernandez Lynch H, Dickert NW, Zettler PJ, et al. Regulatory flexibility for COVID-19 research. J L Biosci 2020;7(1):Isaa057.
13. U.S. Food and Drug Administration. Coronavirus Treatment Acceleration Program (CTAP). 2020. Available at: https://www.fda.gov/drugs/coronavirus-covid-19-drugs/coronavirus-treatment-acceleration-program-ctap. Accessed October 27, 2020.
14. Sathian B, Asim M, Banerjee I, et al. Impact of COVID-19 on clinical trials and clinical research: A systematic review. Nepal J Epidemiol 2020;10(3):878–87.
15. Vidoni ED, Szabo-Reed A, Kang C, et al. The IGNITE trial: Participant recruitment lessons prior to SARS-CoV-2. Contemp Clin Trials Commun 2020;20:100666.
16. Padala PR, Jendro AM, Padala KP. Conducting Clinical Research During the COVID-19 pandemic: investigator and participant perspectives. JMIR Public Health Surveill 2020;6(2):e18887.
17. Davis S, Pai S. Challenges and opportunities for sponsors in conducting clinical trials during a pandemic. Perspect Clin Res 2020;11(3):115–20.
18. McDermott MM, Newman AB. Preserving clinical trial integrity during the coronavirus pandemic. JAMA 2020;323(21):2135–6.

19. van Koningsbruggen-Rietschel S, Dunlevy F, Bulteel V, et al. SARS-CoV-2 disrupts clinical research: the role of a rare disease-specific trial network. Eur Respir J 2020;56(3).

20. Cherry JD. The chronology of the 2002-2003 SARS mini pandemic. Paediatr Respir Rev 2004;5(4):262–9.

21. Teixeira da Silva JA, Tsigaris P, Erfanmanesh M. Publishing volumes in major databases related to Covid-19. Scientometrics 2020;1–12. https://doi.org/10.1007/s11192-020-03675-3.

22. Nowakowska J, Sobocinska J, Lewicki M, et al. When science goes viral: The research response during three months of the COVID-19 outbreak. Biomed Pharmacother 2020;129:110451.

23. Fidahic M, Nujic D, Runjic R, et al. Research methodology and characteristics of journal articles with original data, preprint articles and registered clinical trial protocols about COVID-19. BMC Med Res Methodol 2020;20(1):161.

24. Krumholz HM. The End of Journals. Circ Cardiovasc Qual Outcomes 2015;8(6):533–4.

25. Preprints with The Lancet. Available at: https://www.ssrn.com/index.cfm/en/thelancet/. Accessed October 27, 2020.

26. Flier JS. Covid-19 is reshaping the world of bioscience publishing. First Opinion Web site. 2020. Available at: https://www.statnews.com/2020/03/23/bioscience-publishing-reshaped-covid-19/. Accessed October 27, 2020.

27. Packer M. Does Peer Review Still Matter in the Era of COVID-19?. 2020. Available at: https://www.medpagetoday.com/blogs/revolutionandrevelation/86465. Accessed 16 Oct 2020.

28. Retracted coronavirus (COVID-19) papers. 2020. Available at: https://retractionwatch.com/retracted-coronavirus-covid-19-papers/. Accessed October 27, 2020.

29. Dinis-Oliveira RJ. COVID-19 research: pandemic versus "paperdemic", integrity, values and risks of the "speed science. Forensic Sci Res 2020;5(2):174–87.

30. Ioannidis JPA. Coronavirus disease 2019: the harms of exaggerated information and non-evidence-based measures. Eur J Clin Invest 2020;e13223.

31. Balaphas A, Gkoufa K, Daly MJ, et al. Flattening the curve of new publications on COVID-19. J Epidemiol Community Health 2020;74(9):766–7.

32. London AJ, Kimmelman J. Against pandemic research exceptionalism. Science 2020;368(6490):476–7.

33. Bae S, Kim MC, Kim JY, et al. Effectiveness of Surgical and Cotton Masks in Blocking SARS-CoV-2: A Controlled Comparison in 4 Patients. Ann Intern Med 2020;173(1):W22–3.

34. Mehra MR, Desai SS, Ruschitzka F, et al. RETRACTED: Hydroxychloroquine or chloroquine with or without a macrolide for treatment of COVID-19: a multinational registry analysis. Lancet 2020. https://doi.org/10.1016/S0140-6736(20)31180-6.

35. Funck-Brentano C, Salem JE. Chloroquine or hydroxychloroquine for COVID-19: why might they be hazardous? Lancet 2020. https://doi.org/10.1016/S0140-6736(20)31174-0.

36. Mehra MR, Desai SS, Kuy S, et al. Cardiovascular Disease, Drug Therapy, and Mortality in Covid-19. N Engl J Med 2020;382(25):e102.

37. Lv M, Luo X, Estill J, et al. Coronavirus disease (COVID-19): a scoping review. Euro Surveill 2020;25(15).

38. US National Library of Medicine. Available at: https://clinicaltrials.gov. Accessed October 26, 2020.

39. Keswani SG, Parikh UM, Gosain A, et al. Impact of the coronavirus disease 2019 pandemic on surgical research and lessons for the future. Surgery 2020;169(2): 257–63 [published online ahead of print, 2020 Sep 19].

40. Sharpless NE. COVID-19 and cancer. Science 2020;368(6497):1290.

41. Rosenbaum L. The Untold Toll - The Pandemic's Effects on Patients without Covid-19. N Engl J Med 2020;382(24):2368–71.

42. Bailey C, Black JRM, Swanton C. Cancer research: the lessons to Learn from COVID-19. Cancer Discov 2020;10(9):1263–6.

43. Auletta JJ, Adamson PC, Agin JE, et al. Pediatric cancer research: Surviving COVID-19. Pediatr Blood Cancer 2020;67(9):e28435.

44. Bauchner H, Fontanarosa PB. Randomized Clinical Trials and COVID-19: Managing Expectations. JAMA 2020;323(22):2262–3.

45. Tong A, Elliott JH, Azevedo LC, et al. Core Outcomes Set for Trials in People With Coronavirus Disease 2019. Crit Care Med 2020;48(11):1622–35.

46. Marshall JC, Murthy S, Diaz J, et al. WHO Working Group on the Clinical Characterisation and Management of COVID-19 infection. A minimal common outcome measure set for COVID-19 clinical research. Lancet Infect Dis 2020;20(8):e192–7 [published correction appears in Lancet Infect Dis 2020;20(10):e250].

47. WhiteHouse.gov. Open Acces Letter from CSAs. 2020. Available at: https://www. whitehouse.gov/wp-content/uploads/2020/03/COVID19-Open-Access-Letter-from-CSAs.Equivalents-Final.pdf. Accessed October 28, 2020.

48. Navar AM, Pencina MJ, Rymer JA, et al. Use of Open Access Platforms for Clinical Trial Data. JAMA 2016;315(12):1283–4.

49. Price-Haywood EG, Burton J, Fort D, et al. Hospitalization and mortality among black patients and white patients with covid-19. N Engl J Med 2020;382(26): 2534–43.

50. Laurencin CT, McClinton A. The COVID-19 Pandemic: a Call to Action to Identify and Address Racial and Ethnic Disparities. J Racial Ethn Health Disparities 2020; 7(3):398–402.

51. Kabarriti R, Brodin NP, Maron MI, et al. Association of Race and Ethnicity With Comorbidities and Survival Among Patients With COVID-19 at an Urban Medical Center in New York. JAMA Netw Open 2020;3(9):e2019795.

52. Massachusetts General Hospital. COVID-19 ICU REGISTRY: A Multicenter International Data Repository. Available at: https://www.massgeneral.org/anesthesia/ research/covid-19-icu-registry. Accessed October 31, 2020.

53. RED CORAL: PETAL Repository of Electronic Data COVID-19 Observational Study. Available at: https://petalnet.org/studies/public/redcoral. Accessed October 31, 2020.

54. El-Boghdadly K, Wong DJN, Owen R, et al. Risks to healthcare workers following tracheal intubation of patients with COVID-19: a prospective international multicentre cohort study. Anaesthesia 2020;75(11):1437–47.

55. Stock AD, Bader ER, Cezayirli P, et al. COVID-19 Infection Among Healthcare Workers: Serological Findings Supporting Routine Testing. Front Med (Lausanne) 2020;7:471.

56. Buitrago-Garcia D, Egli-Gany D, Counotte MJ, et al. Occurrence and transmission potential of asymptomatic and presymptomatic SARS-CoV-2 infections: A living systematic review and meta-analysis. PLoS Med 2020;17(9):e1003346.

Moving?

Make sure your subscription moves with you!

To notify us of your new address, find your **Clinics Account Number** (located on your mailing label above your name), and contact customer service at:

Email: journalscustomerservice-usa@elsevier.com

800-654-2452 (subscribers in the U.S. & Canada)
314-447-8871 (subscribers outside of the U.S. & Canada)

Fax number: 314-447-8029

Elsevier Health Sciences Division
Subscription Customer Service
3251 Riverport Lane
Maryland Heights, MO 63043

*To ensure uninterrupted delivery of your subscription, please notify us at least 4 weeks in advance of move.

ELSEVIER

Printed and bound by CPI Group (UK) Ltd, Croydon, CR0 4YY

08/05/2025

01864700-0005